The Joseph H. Pilates

Method at Home

A balance, shape, strength, & fitness program

ELEANOR McKENZIE
TREVOR BLOUNT

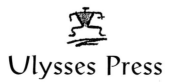

Ulysses Press

Published in the United States by
Ulysses Press
P.O. Box 3440
Berkeley, CA 94703
www.ulyssespress.com

Interior Designer Rozelle Bentheim
Cover Designer Sarah Levin
Special Photography Mark Winwood
Model Katarina Thome
Scientific Illustration Philip Wilson

Distributed in the United States
by Publishers Group West and
in Canada by Raincoast Books

First published in Great Britain in 2000 by Hamlyn,
a division of Octopus Publishing Group Limited,
2–4 Heron Quays, Docklands, London, E14 4JP.

Copyright © 2000 Octopus Publishing Group Ltd.

ISBN 1-56975-210-9

Library of Congress Card Number 99-69193

Printed in Hong Kong

It is advisable to check with your doctor
before embarking on any exercise
program. The Joseph H. Pilates Method
should not be considered a replacement
for professional medical treatment; a
physician should be consulted in all
matters relating to health and
particularly in respect of pregnancy and
any symptoms that may require
diagnosis or medical attention. While
the advice and information in this book
is believed to be accurate and the step-
by-step instructions have been devised
to avoid strain, neither the author nor
the publisher can accept any legal
responsibility for any injury sustained
while following the exercises.

contents

The Joseph H. Pilates Method at Home

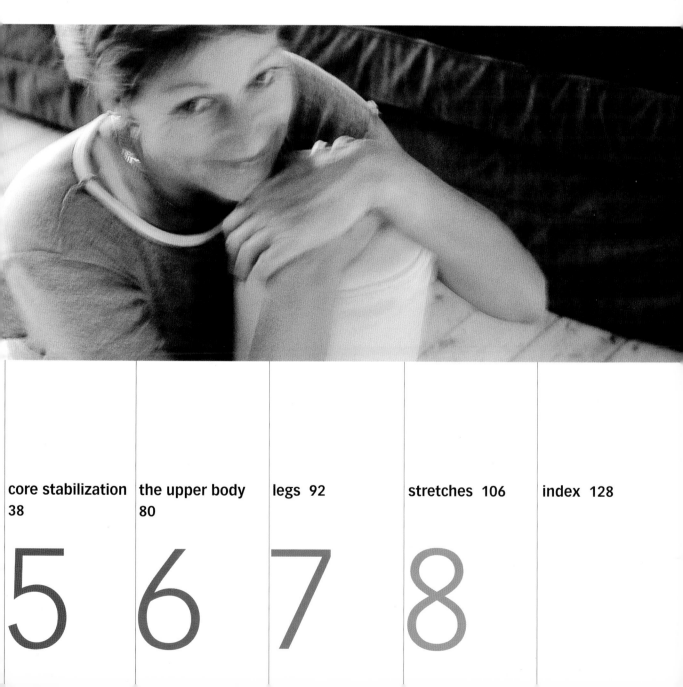

Pilates has recently enjoyed an explosion of popularity but its success is based not on a transient whim of fashion, but rather on the positive experiences of the people who have benefited from Pilates first-hand. Gone were their backaches, sore necks and strained muscles – Pilates had re-educated their bodies to work in a way sympathetic to their anatomy.

This book deals with one aspect of Pilates, the fundamental principle that underpins all Pilates exercises, core stabilization. It is a collection of exercises, which focus on the torso and build inner muscular strength. This group of muscles then gives stability to move the limbs efficiently and safely. To gain the most benefit from Pilates, it is essential to instil the principles of core stabilization in your mind and body. Only then will you be ready for more challenging Pilates. Even when performing the most advanced Pilates exercises, you will find your mind, like a never-ending circle, refocusing on the principles of core stabilization.

This book is my view of Pilates, a view I have formed through fifteen years of my own daily practise and teaching. I have taught, together with many other dedicated Pilates instructors,

foreword

people of all ages and walks of life. All of these people have been my teachers. Through them I have learnt that Pilates is a way of re-educating our minds and bodies.

Thought is the key, every movement in Pilates is deliberate and demands concentration. This act of will fuses mind and body and gives the feeling of well-being characteristic of regular Pilates. If you keep yourself strong and flexible and you are aware of your body through your experience of Pilates, you will be less likely to suffer injuries and postural problems, and if you do, you will recover more quickly. Regular practice is essential because the truth about the quick fix is that it just doesn't exist. Real and lasting change happens over time.

This focus on core stabilization sets this book apart from any other on the market and also makes it the most effective, because it paves the ways for maximum benefit when you attempt more challenging Pilates exercises. The emphasis is placed on the process and experience of practice. If you focus on this, you will enjoy your Pilates, and gain real and lasting benefits, just as I and many other people have done. **Trevor Blount**

'It doesn't matter what you do, it's the way that you do it.'

Joseph H. Pilates

The modern world is constructed in order to maximize leisure time and minimize physical activity. Exercise that in the past was an integral part of life, such as walking and household tasks requiring physical exertion, has been supplanted by machines and cars. Many changes in the last 20 years have ensured that at home and at work we exercise our bodies as little as possible.

Since we do not walk as much or perform other physically strenuous tasks, we now need to take conscious steps to ensure that we exercise our bodies in our leisure time. We often hope that the relaxation that comes from our leisure time will release us from the constant strain of life's demands and bring relief from the tension in both our minds and our bodies. However, what we commonly mean by relaxation is lying in bed or watching television, neither of which offers true relaxation to the body or mind.

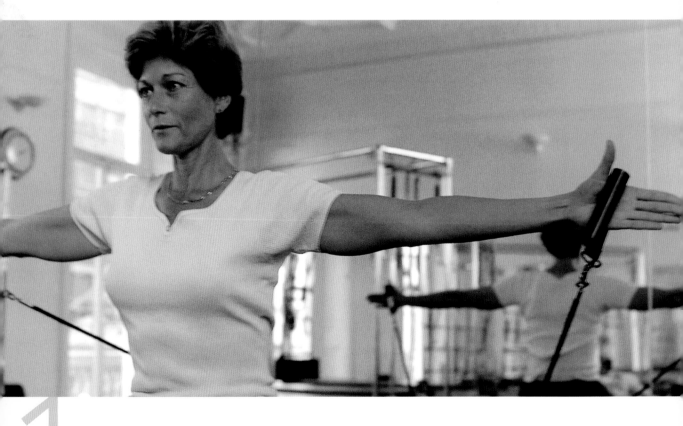

pilates: history and philosophy

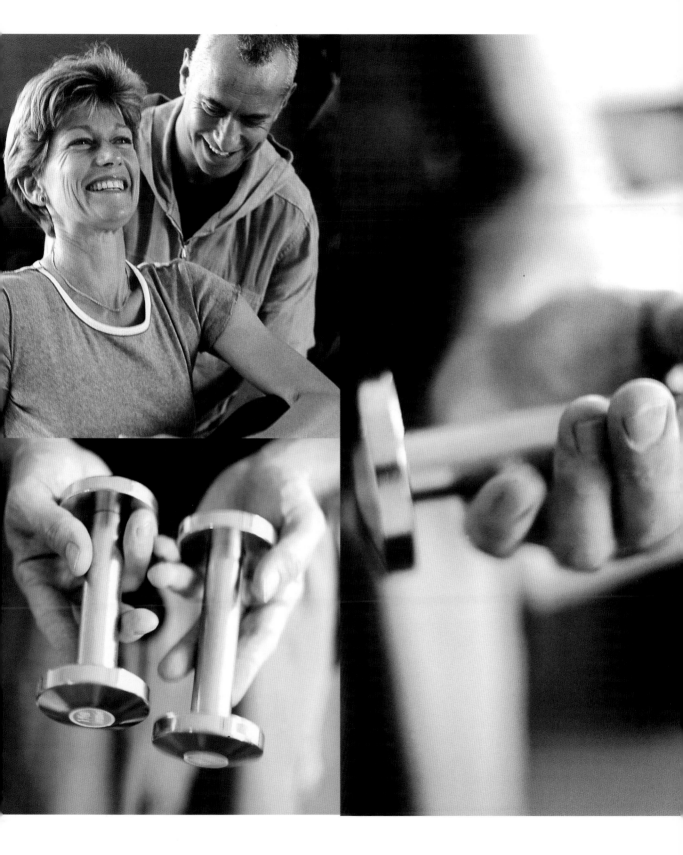

The origins of Pilates

Pilates (pronounced pih-lah-teez) is a modern system of body maintenance named after its inventor, Joseph H. Pilates. Originally, Pilates called it Contrology, but it is now commonly known as Pilates. Pilates defined Contrology as the complete coordination of body, mind and spirit. In this respect it differs from other modern forms of physical exercise such as aerobics as it aims to be holistic in its approach to physical fitness.

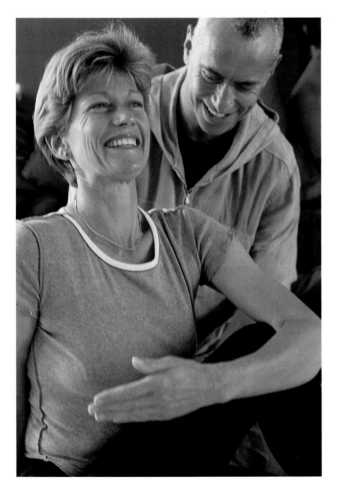

The life of Joseph Pilates

Joseph Pilates was born in Germany in 1880. As a child he suffered from asthma, rickets and rheumatic fever, and it was these childhood illnesses that drove him to discover a method of overcoming them. He focused on sports as one way of building physical strength, and became a skilled gymnast and talented skier, as well as a boxer and a wrestler. At the same time he became passionately interested in human physiology, especially the musculature of the body. He studied this alongside forms of exercise from the East, such as yoga. It was the combination of all these interests that led him to devise Contrology.

In 1912, Joseph Pilates moved to England, where he had a varied career as a boxer, a circus performer and a self-defence instructor. The outbreak of war between Britain and Germany in 1914 interrupted this career. As a German national, he was interned for the duration of the war along with other fellow countrymen who were living in Britain at the time. However, it was this experience that was to lead him to fully develop his own method for achieving physical fitness.

Confined in the prison camp he devised exercises to keep himself and his fellow internees healthy. He used beds and other pieces of furniture to construct the prototypes of the equipment seen in Pilates studios today. He later claimed that these exercises protected the internees from the flu epidemic of 1918 that killed thousands in Britain, and from other illnesses that often resulted from living in confined, crowded conditions.

pilates: history and philosophy

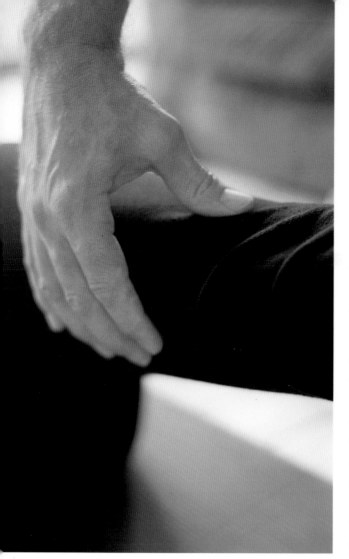

On his voyage to America he met a nurse, Clara, with whom he spent the journey discussing health and the importance of keeping the body healthy. By the end of the journey they had decided to open a physical fitness studio together, which they did in the same building as the New York City Ballet. Later they also married.

As in Germany, Pilates attracted many of the top dancers because his method of exercising complemented the dancer's traditional training. Soon actors, actresses and sports people, as well as wealthy socialites, were hurrying to Pilates' studio to learn his unique method of strengthening the body without building a bulky musculature.

Today, Pilates has become popular worldwide. It is practised by people from all backgrounds, although it still has a particular appeal for dancers, actors and other physical performers, who use it as part of their professional training, rather than just as a means of keeping fit. Pilates' philosophy of physical fitness has something to offer everyone, regardless of age and physical ability, particularly those who would like strength and tone without building huge muscles.

Pilates' philosophy of physical fitness

Fundamental to Pilates' philosophy was the idea that elements of civilization were detrimental to physical fitness. He believed that the modern lifestyle caused stress-related illnesses, with telephones, cars, economic pressure and environmental pollution all combining to create physical and mental stress. Pilates further

On his release from the camp at the end of the war he returned to Germany, where he continued to develop his method. Then he met a man who was to be very influential in the world of modern dance, Rudolf von Laban, who was the inventor of a method of dance notation called Labanotation. Von Laban incorporated some of Pilates' exercises into his teaching, as have other famous dance innovators such as Hanya Holm, Martha Graham and George Balanchine.

His techniques attracted not only dancers, but also the Hamburg police force, whom he spent some time training. However, in 1926, when he was ordered rather than asked to train the new German army, he immediately left for America.

claimed that this stress was so overwhelming that every household probably had at least one person who suffered from nervous tension. His theories were ahead of his time, and have now been widely proved.

To relieve the effects of daily stress, Pilates believed, people needed a reserve of energy in order to allow them to participate in diverse forms of recreational activity, preferably outdoors. To Pilates the concept of play was crucial in the fight against stress, but he realized that most people were so tired after work that they considered an evening of reading the paper to be the only leisure activity they could manage.

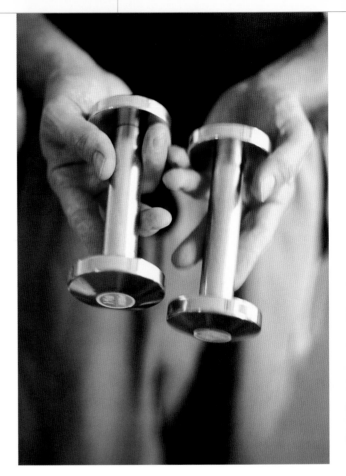

He also believed that people entered a cycle of stress and tension that was difficult to break. He illustrated this point by describing the effects of a brief holiday. Ideally, a break from a familiar routine and environment should have the effect of revitalizing us. However, Pilates said, the levels of mental and physical strain suffered by many people meant that they did not have the necessary energy reserves to cope with a change in environment, and so instead of feeling revitalized they became even more stressed. This, he emphasized, was not a natural response, but one induced by the strains of modern daily life. Today there are numerous articles on the stresses of taking a holiday and the inability of some people to relax while away – they say holidays make them feel worse than when they are at work. Moreover, during a holiday, relationship or family tensions are bound to arise as people suddenly find themselves together in a strange environment for days or weeks at a time.

In order to respond naturally to life and the changes and stresses it involves, Pilates recognized that we need to be physically and mentally fit. Trauma and stress are less likely to affect people who feel well in mind and body and who are aware of what they can do to offset the negative effects of stressful events. Physical fitness is a useful attribute when coping with stress. Tired people often react to stressful events in such a way as to create more stress for themselves. Physical fatigue takes its toll on mental alertness, making it harder to function efficiently. The relationship between physical and mental fatigue is unquestionable.

In his book *Return to Life Through Contrology*, Pilates explained that physical fitness is the attainment and maintenance of a uniformly developed body with a sound mind capable of naturally and satisfactorily performing varied daily tasks with spontaneous zest

pilates: history and philosophy

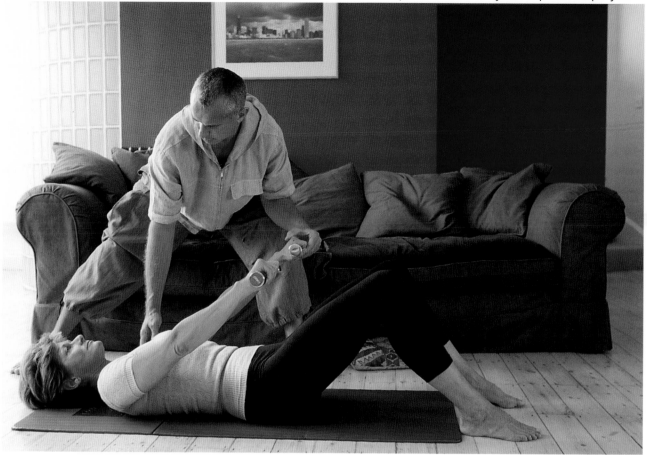

and pleasure. To compete in the modern world we need to be fit, but we cannot buy fitness like a new car, or acquire it just by thinking about it; we have to take action with our bodies, and, in the case of Pilates, with our minds as well. The improved health of both of these will in turn affect the spirit.

The essence of Pilates

What differentiates Pilates from other forms of exercise is primarily its holistic approach and its combined training of mind and body to achieve correct postural alignment. Pilates considers the entire body, rather than targeting problem areas. When practising Pilates it is also important to remember that the process is more important than the result – the aim is not to achieve a culturally accepted body but rather one which is naturally aligned.

The key elements of Pilates:

- lengthening short muscles and strengthening weak muscles
- improving the quality of movement
- focusing on the core postural muscles to stabilize the body
- working to place the breath correctly
- controlling even the smallest movements
- understanding and improving good body mechanics
- mental relaxation

The mechanical system that allows us to move – to walk, run and jump – is dependent on the harmonious relationship between our skeleton and our voluntary muscles.

One of the main functions of our voluntary muscles is to protect our skeleton. Unlike involuntary muscles, such as the pupil of the eye, we are able to control our voluntary muscles. We constantly send these muscles messages via the brain, telling them to perform specific actions.

As we get older we are often amazed to find that our muscles no longer do exactly what we want. We know that the machines we use need to be looked after. In a similar way, we must develop an awareness of our bodies as organisms that need to be cared for if we don't want them to break down.

Pilates takes this further and stresses the need for mindful exercise. By controlling our movements, we link mind and body, a concept which is fundamental to Pilates.

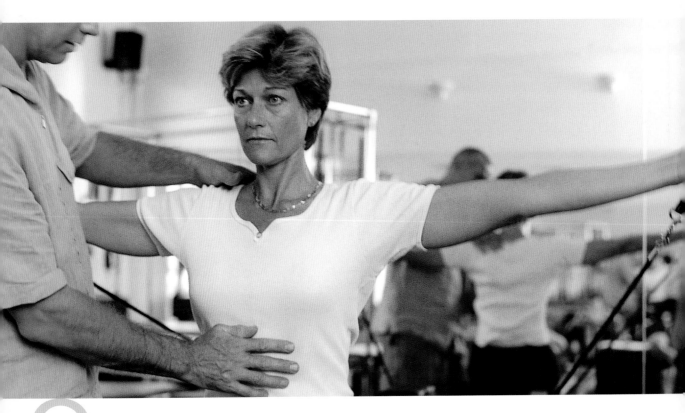

2 the musculo-skeletal body

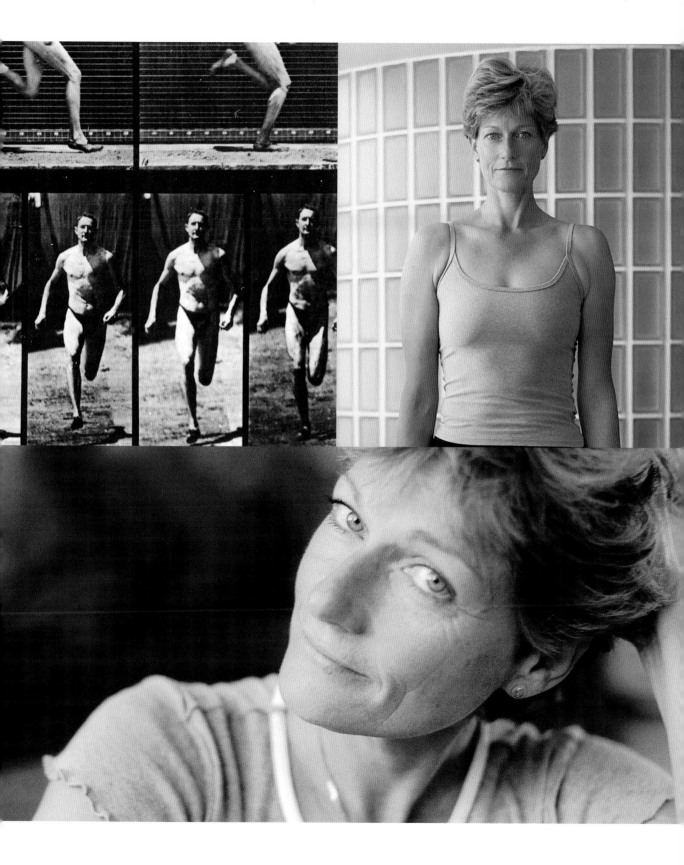

The muscle theory

When Pilates propounded his theory, his principal aim was to develop the body uniformly. He was aware that people often had 'pet' sets of muscles they wanted to work on. For example, some people are concerned with having a flat stomach and so exercise only their stomach muscles. Pilates was determined to emphasize that this would not promote total muscle health, or indeed total overall health, as good muscle tone is necessary to keep all the internal organs in condition and in their proper place.

With Pilates you will gain control of your entire body. The repetition of the exercises and performance of them in a mindful way will gradually allow you to acquire a natural coordination of your muscles that is normally associated with subconscious activities.

Pilates wrote that all animals have this natural coordination and control. Watch a cat wake up; instead of leaping up, it stretches all its muscles before it moves. Pilates may have taken this element of his theory from Eastern practices. Those who do yoga, chi kung or tai chi will be aware that many postures are named after animals because they are based on the movements of those particular animals. The aim behind the imitation of animal movements is that the person will acquire the balance, suppleness and strength of these animals, as well as their health and vitality.

Normally, in childhood we have a naturally relaxed posture, but as we mature our bodies start to reflect the strains of life. We acquire incorrect posture without noticing that it is happening, and this in turn filters through to other physical functions and depletes our vitality. Some posture problems arise as a result of one's occupation: any work that requires the repetitive use of particular sets of muscles results in postural imbalance. This may be sedentary work which encourages poor sitting posture, or, for example, hairdressing or other work that requires people to stand for long periods of time, placing undue stress on specific parts of the body.

Other postural problems can have an emotional basis. People who carry an emotional burden can often be seen to literally carry it on their shoulders, which have physically bent under the weight. Finally, some postural problems are inherited.

Pilates not only helps to correct your postural problems; it also aims to give you mastery of your mind. Joseph Pilates was convinced that lack of regular, conscious exercise also caused a deterioration in brain function. His theory is based partly in physiology and partly in philosophy. The first part of Pilates' theory states that the brain is comparable to a telephone switchboard that controls communication between the sympathetic nervous system and the muscles. He then went on to say that many of our daily activities are performed on the basis of what we THINK we see, hear or touch, without considering the positive or negative results of our actions. This leads to the formation of habit and automatic actions. In Pilates' theory, the ideal condition is that our muscles should obey our will, and

the musculo-skeletal body

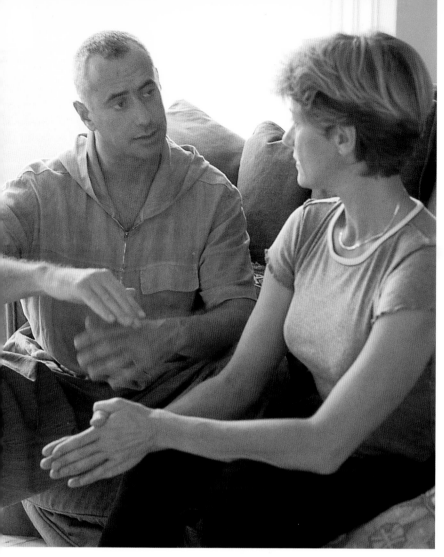

Muscle memory

One aspect of the relationship between the mind and muscles is muscle memory. This plays a key part in learning any new exercise, but is particularly important in understanding Pilates, as the central aim of the exercises is re-education of the body, a large part of which is re-education of the muscle memory. Muscles memorize particular movements, especially frequently repeated movements carried out over a long period. Once these movements have been firmly implanted in the memory functions of both muscle and mind, it is very difficult to change

that our will should not be dominated by our reflex actions. In this Pilates was strongly influenced by the German philosopher Schopenhauer.

Put simply, Joseph Pilates believed that we perform physical movements without conscious thought and that this is not good for either mind or body. Conscious movement, on the other hand, uses brain cells, which prevents them from dying, and this in turn helps to enhance the activity of the mind. This, Pilates believed, was what accounted for the feeling of uplift in spirits that followed the regular practice of his exercises, which steadily increased the supply of blood to the brain and thereby stimulated areas that had previously been dormant.

them. For example, if you work at a desk you will have a particular way of sitting. It is uniquely your way of sitting. Trying to change your usual sitting posture for any length of time will cause you discomfort because your muscles want to return to the position to which they are accustomed. Also, the moment you take your attention away from the new posture, your body will automatically return to the old one. That is why Pilates places so much emphasis on mindfulness or conscious exercise, because it is when you lose focus on what your body and muscles are doing that your body does what it feels like, not what you want it to do.

Working the muscles three ways

Pilates emphasizes working the muscles through the three dimensions. The reason for this is that if you work the muscle in only one dimension the other two remain tight. For example, if you are working on stretching the hamstrings, the muscle is first exercised with the leg in the natural parallel position. The stretch is repeated with the leg rotated out, then rotated in (see pages 110–111). This ensures that all dimensions of the muscle group are worked on.

Types of muscle movement

Muscle size is not important, but condition is. Muscles can easily become weak and tight, but by working them, using the following three types of muscle contraction, they can be strengthened and lengthened. This also improves the condition of the muscles and joints. It is also vital to learn to exercise in a relaxed way, reducing tension and allowing the body's movements to flow. Athletes perfect examples of this. Just before a race an athlete focuses on relaxation, since good results depend on freedom of movement. Sometimes less is more.

The three types of muscle contraction are:

1. Isometric
2. Concentric
3. Eccentric

Isometric contraction (below) is static. Tension is developed in the muscle without the joint being moved. See pages 46–47 for the complete exercise.

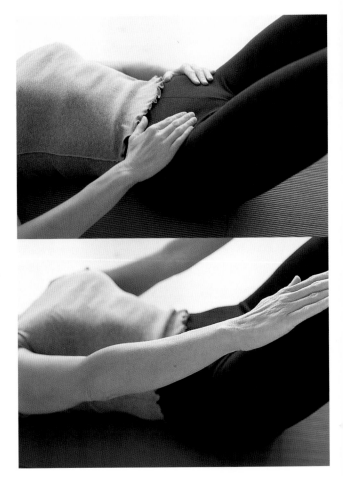

the musculo-skeletal body

Concentric contraction (below) occurs when the muscle is shortened in movement. This is usual in conventional exercises, such as abdominal crunches. See pages 54–55 for the complete exercise.

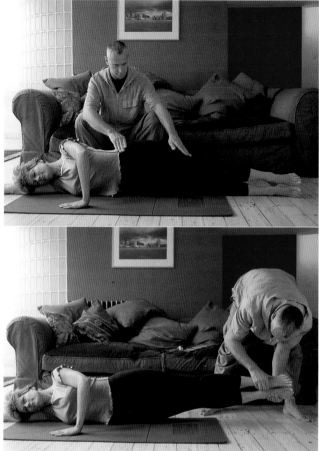

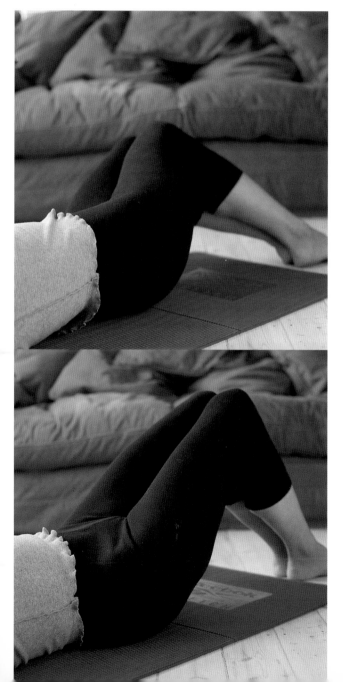

Eccentric contraction (above) lengthens muscles. This movement should not to be confused with stretching, as you can not contract a muscle and stretch it at the same time. It is eccentric muscle contraction that is strongly emphasized in Pilates. See pages 58–59 for the complete exercise.

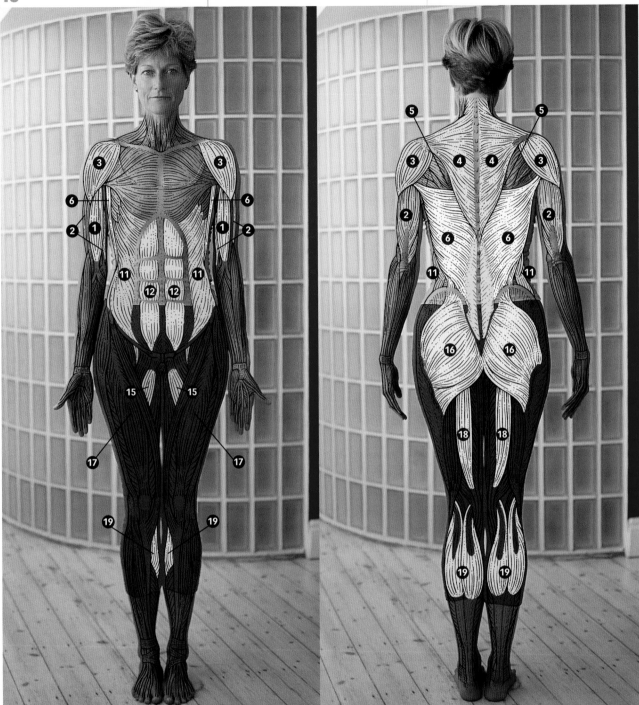

Important muscles

Muscles generate movement by pulling on the tendons that are attached to the bones. Most body movements involve more than one group of muscles. Movement is also created by a pair of muscles working in opposition to each other – one muscle moves the joint in one direction while the other muscle pulls the joint back. There are hundreds of muscles in the body that can be consciously controlled. You do not need to know all of them. However, it is useful to know the names and the actions of the main muscles focused on in Pilates.

the musculo-skeletal body

1. Biceps – front of the upper arm, used to move the arm.

2. Triceps – back of upper arm, used to move the arm.

3. Deltoid – encloses the shoulder and upper arm, used to move the arm backwards and forwards.

4. Trapezius – runs down the back of the neck and along the shoulders, used to extend the head.

5. Rhomboid – attaches the shoulder blades to the spine. Most of it lies beneath the Trapezius muscle.

6. Latissimus dorsi – popularly referred to as 'lats', it runs from the lower chest into the lumbar region. It pulls the shoulders down and back and the body upwards.

7. Erector spinae – (not shown) found at the back of the neck, chest and abdomen. This important muscle extends the spine and holds the body upright.

8. Quadratus lumborum – (not shown) deep interior waist muscle.

9. Transversus abdominis – (not shown) deep internal muscle that runs across the abdomen. It applies pressure to the abdomen and holds the organs in place. It lies beneath the internal oblique muscle.

10. Internal oblique – (not shown) horizontally crosses the abdomen, compresses the abdomen and moves the trunk. It lies beneath the external oblique muscle.

11. External oblique – side muscle of the abdomen. It compresses the abdomen and is used when moving the trunk in any direction.

12. Rectus abdominis – popularly known as the 'abs', this muscle runs vertically down the entire front of the abdomen. This postural muscle draws the front of the pelvis upwards.

13. Perineum – (not shown) an internal muscle. It forms the pelvic floor and attaches to the pelvic wall which is located deep in the pelvic cavity.

14. Psoas – (not shown) also known as hip flexor. This is a deep muscle which runs from the front of the femur to the lumbar region of the spine.

15. Adductor – an inner thigh muscle, used for moving the leg inward.

16. Gluteus maximus – forms the buttocks. It is used for running and jumping.

17. Quadriceps extensor – runs down the middle of the front of the thigh. It performs the opposite movement to the hamstrings.

18. Semitendinosus – also known as the hamstrings. It runs down the middle of the back of the thigh. Used to extend the thigh and to flex the leg at the knee joint.

19. Gastrocnemius – forms the greater part of the calf. This muscle runs down the back of the lower leg.

There are more than 600 skeletal muscles in your body. In total, they account for 35–50 per cent of your body mass. With their partners, the ligaments and tendons, your body's muscles perform two main functions:

1. Muscles provide you with your basic stability. For instance, the muscles of the back support your spinal column the way rigging supports a yacht mast. They give your spine stability when subjected to strong external forces, such as when lifting a heavy load.

2. Muscles are used for performing tasks (walking, lifting, pulling and so on). The process begins with a message travelling from the brain, down the spinal cord to a spinal nerve root, and then out along that nerve to the appropriate muscles. The message tells your muscles what to do and how to do it.

Injuries to the back occur more often in the muscles than in the skeleton or nerves because muscles are under the greatest amount of daily stress. Back muscles work constantly to provide support for your spine. If your muscles are weak or underdeveloped, almost any activity can result in a muscle strain or tear, and that carries with it the added risk of damage to a vertebra, nerve or disc.

The greatest risk of muscle injury comes when you use your back (and the surrounding) muscles to perform unusually strenuous work. Their ability to undertake any given task without injury depends on their strength and flexibility. However, the technique you use when performing the task is even more important.

You cannot do much about the bones and the nerves you were born with, but you can do something about your muscle development, body weight and general fitness. You can also improve your understanding of good posture and the way your body's mechanics work.

1. **Cervical vertebrae** – this section of the spine, the top seven vertebrae, is very flexible and allows the head a large range of movement. However, It is this flexibility that makes the cervical spine particularly vulnerable to injury.

2. **Thoracic vertebrae** – these twelve vertebrae articulate with the twelve pairs of ribs.

3. **Lumbar vertebrae** – the five vertebrae between the ribs and pelvis are known as the powerhouse of the spine as they bear the weight of the torso.

4. **Sacral vertebrae** – these five vertebrae are fused together with the Coccyx to make solid bone.

5. **Coccyx** – the bottom four vertebrae of the spine.

6. **Sternum** – this links with the top ten pairs of ribs, leaving the two lowest pairs floating.

7. **Ribs** – these form a protective cage which shield the internal organs from injury.

8. **Pelvis** – this strong structure is made up of three fused bones; the wing-shaped ilium; the pubis in front; and the ischium behind.

the musculo-skeletal body

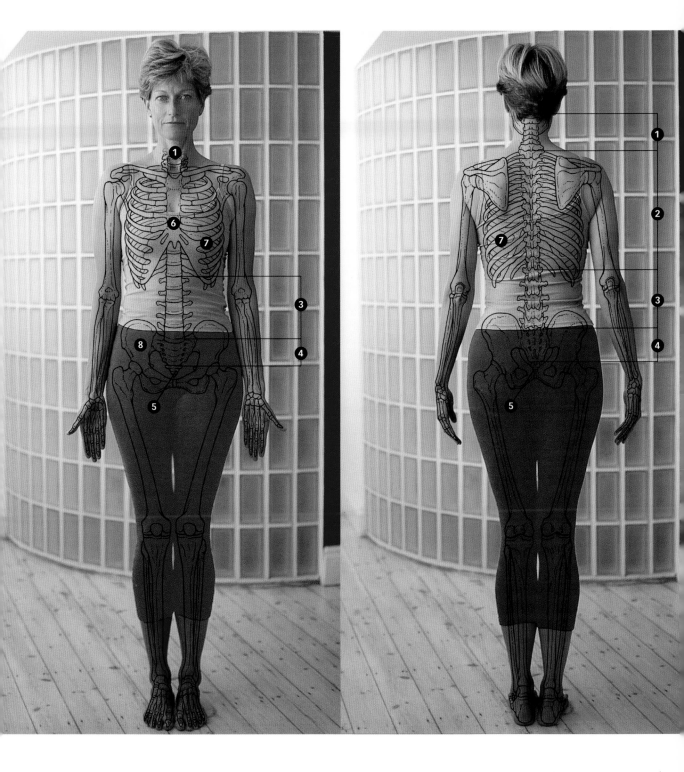

Most of us try a new method of treatment or exercise because we are looking for a cure for one specific problem. If we decide on a form of bodywork, such as Pilates, it is often because we have a musculo-skeletal problem. We could be suffering from a recurring back complaint that is the result of an accident in earlier years, or a congenital condition that causes a deformity of the spine, such as scoliosis (see page 34), or a work-related problem, such as repetitive strain injury (RSI).

However, the Pilates teacher will not only look at your primary problem; they will ask you questions about your medical history and your lifestyle, and assess your mental and emotional make-up. The teacher will then look at your posture, assessing where you hold tension and where there is an imbalance. It is only after all this information has been gathered and assessed that the Pilates teacher will create an exercise programme that is tailor-made for you and the condition of your body.

3 the teacher's eye

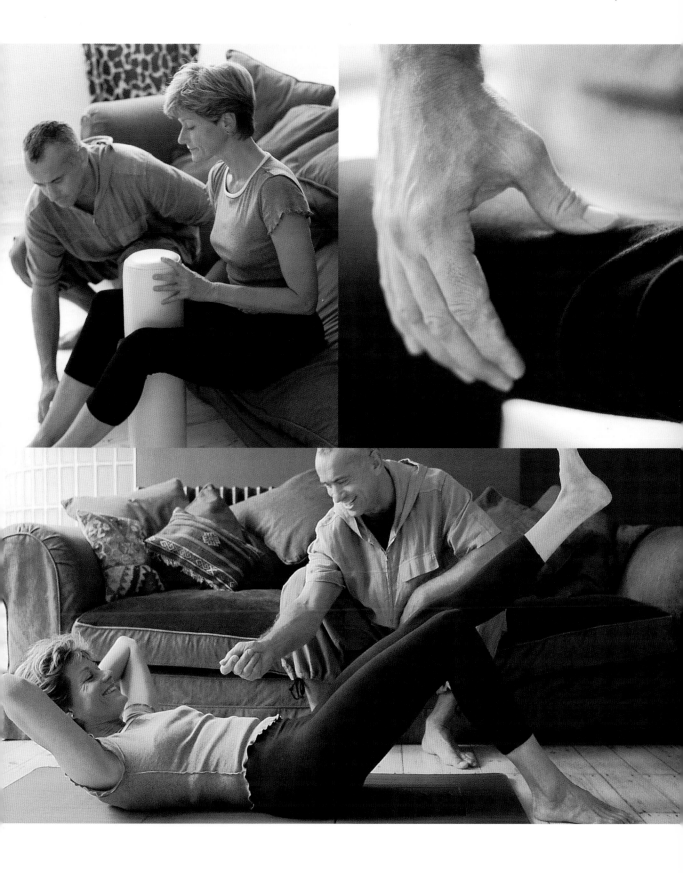

Selecting a teacher

This book is a source of self-help, but instruction from a teacher will take you beyond anything that you can teach yourself. For example, you can teach yourself to play tennis or golf, but if you go to a coach you will learn things you could not have taught yourself. For a start, the coach can look at you objectively, which you can't. They also have an experienced eye that can spot where minor changes in technique will have a major effect. In Pilates, where precision of movement is fundamental, only the eye of an experienced teacher can see where you are going wrong and make the necessary adjustments.

As with other therapies, you need to find a teacher with whom you feel comfortable and who has a good understanding of you and your physical condition. You may find the right person immediately, or have to try several before you find someone with whom you feel happy to work. Personal recommendation is a good way to start.

It is also important to find a teacher who has had the correct training. Pilates training takes two years. Those who have undertaken this are accredited by the PilatesFoundation, which was founded in 1996 and is an independent, non-profit-making organization governing Pilates teachers in the UK and Europe. Searching the Internet will also provide you with information about teachers, their studios and their philosophy.

Where to practise

The ideal place to practise is at a teacher's studio, but as these are often found only in major cities, you may have no choice but to practise at home. In this case, you may be able to find a teacher who will come to your home to instruct you, just as a personal trainer would. The only shortcoming of working at home, with or without a teacher, is that you will not have access to the equipment that is used in a studio.

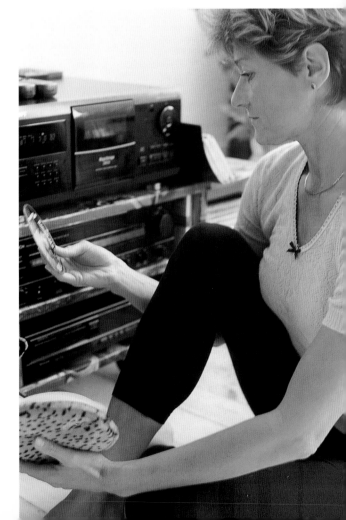

the teacher's eye

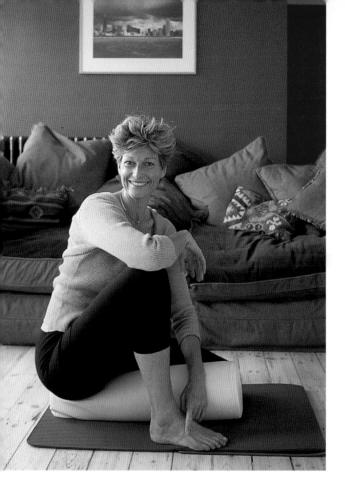

When you choose to practise is up to you. Some people believe that it is better to exercise later in the day because the muscles have already been warmed up. On the other hand, by waiting until later you may get so caught up in daily activities that you decide to postpone your exercise session until tomorrow, then the day after that and so on. The Core Stabilization exercise plan shown in this book warms up the muscles anyway, so that there is no need to perform a separate warm-up routine, as with other forms of exercise. So if you are the type of person who is able to get up early and exercise before work, that is a good time to do it – before the day takes you over.

Practising at home

Pilates exercises require you to be totally focused on what you are doing. For this reason you should always aim to exercise in a place and at a time when you can be sure you will not be disturbed by people or noises, such as the telephone ringing. This does not mean that you have to exercise in total silence – you can play calming music.

You will also need to make a space in which to do the exercises. If you are fortunate enough to be able to devote one room to your Pilates, that will save you from having to clear an area every time you want to practise. If not, find an area in your home that can be used without you having to move half the furniture around before you are able to start, otherwise you will be discouraged.

You will not require any special clothing, just wear something light and comfortable that does not restrict your movement, and is preferably made of natural fibres, which will keep you cooler. Make sure the room is warm enough, as your muscles will automatically tense if you feel cold.

Equipment

The exercises in this book are purposely limited to those you can do at home with the minimum of equipment. Most exercises will be done lying on the floor, and so you will need an exercise mat, which you can get from most sports equipment shops. Alternatively, you can use a blanket folded lengthways, but it should also be wide enough to allow for some movement from side to side. Do not work on a carpet,

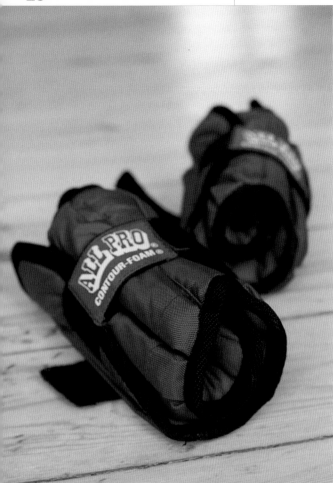

hand weights. These should be 1–1.5kg (2lb 4oz–3lb 5oz) a pair. Older people should choose the lighter weight first, whereas a younger, fitter person can use the 1.5kg (3lb 5oz) weight immediately. These too can be bought from a sports shop. You will find that it is better to use weights rather than cans or bags of rice, as they do not provide the same comfort or ease in performing the movements. You can also buy ankle weights, which will boost the effects of resistance in some of the leg exercises.

Pilates studio equipment

The exercises in this book consist entirely of the mat-work type that can be done at home. In a Pilates studio you will find equipment based on the pieces which Joseph Pilates constructed when he was interned during World War II. They add resistance to the exercises, and so help you to improve your ability to control your body.

as it is not sufficient to protect your spine from being bruised, and is uncomfortable anyway. Also, do not practise on a bed, as it is too soft.

For some exercises you will need a pillow or cushion. Also, people with neck problems might want to put a folded towel or small pillow under their neck for support. This will be indicated at the relevant exercises. A few of the exercises require the use of light

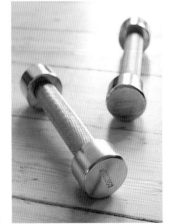

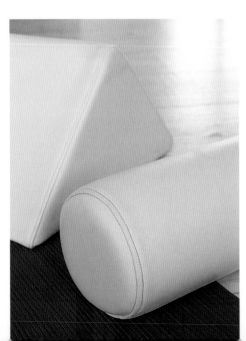

the teacher's eye

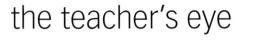

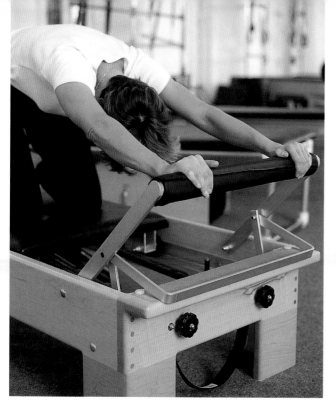

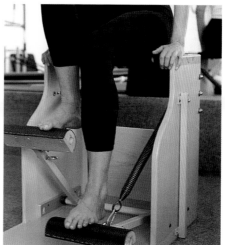

The Reformer

This multi-functional piece of equipment uses tension springs to add resistance. It provides a means of working the entire body through strengthening and lengthening the muscles. However, unlike the weight machines found in a conventional gym, it builds strength without building bulk.

The Cadillac

In a studio, many of the exercises in this book would be performed on this piece of equipment, but at home these exercises may be done on a mat. The Cadillac has specialized attachments for working on spinal articulation and muscle strength. There are many advanced exercises that involve using the Cadillac, but these can be acrobatic and take years to perfect.

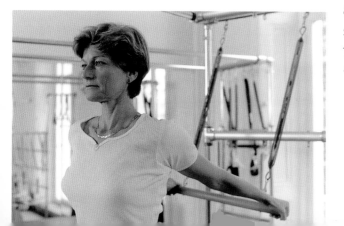

The Chair

This may be the original step machine, and it has the ability to work the whole body. It is a very advanced piece of equipment because it requires you to support your entire body weight while using it, as opposed to the other pieces of equipment that partially support your body while you perform the exercises.

Exercise duration

If you are going to a studio, you are advised to try and attend twice a week, although teachers are aware that this ideal is not possible for everyone. Sessions at a studio usually last one and a half hours.

If you do Pilates at home, you will need to be realistic about how much time you have to exercise daily. You should be honest about your approach to exercise. Trainers at a health club recently identified a number of 'work-out personalities'. One is the 'sporadic achiever'.

Such people start by practising fanatically. They practise every day, possibly several times a day if they are able. They set themselves unrealistic targets, and when they realize they are not going to attain them they stop exercising altogether. This stop-start approach means that they never see any real results. Regularity is essential. Remember that you are trying to re-educate the body and the muscle memory, and that this is more likely to happen if you remind the body every day, even if only for a short time, rather than expecting it to remember what you did seven days ago.

When you are learning the exercises it will take you longer to complete the entire exercise plan. The most important thing is to do the exercises properly. Ideally you should aim for two sessions of one and a half hours per week, and if you can do 15–30 minutes every day in addition to this, that is a bonus. On days when you have less time, do more exercises but fewer repetitions. This is better than doing fewer exercises and keeping the repetitions at the maximum amount, as you will still be working the whole body rather than just one part of it.

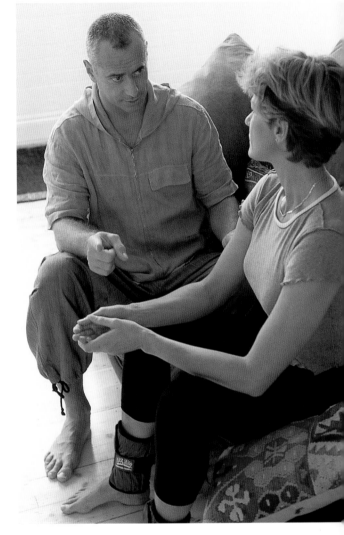

The Pilates method emphasizes mindfulness. You do not simply perform the exercises as actions only. You must concentrate on following the movements precisely, and at the same time be aware of what you are experiencing physically. This is the opposite of most conventional exercises, which require frequent repetition of actions without focus on whole body awareness.

Additionally, in Pilates, the number of repetitions of an exercise is deliberately low, the maximum number being ten at the most, while some must not exceed five repetitions. The reasoning behind this is that if you are performing an exercise accurately, you will feel the muscle working. If you then keep repeating the exercise you will work the muscle to exhaustion. This is to be avoided, because when a muscle is tired you stop working it and instead you build up tension in other muscles, which in turn means you start using the wrong muscles.

the teacher's eye

Times to avoid exercise

As with most forms of exercise, there are times when you should not try to practise.

– Do not exercise if you are feeling unwell. You will not benefit from exercise at this time as you will be unable to focus correctly on what you are doing. Instead, you should concentrate on using your energy to get better. You could use your exercise time to do meditation or creative visualization. Alternatively, run a hot bath and add some aromatherapy oils. If it is a very hot bath you should stay in it for 5–15 minutes only. The heat of a hot bath brings toxins to the surface of the skin. Follow this with a shower to rinse off the toxins. Take very hot baths only if you do not have to go out again, as they make you drowsy and activate a sweating action some hours later. If you do not like hot baths, take a warm one that in which you can relax. Again you will benefit from adding oils or mineral salts, which help to relax the muscles and draw out toxins.

– If you are pregnant you should consult an experienced Pilates teacher before you exercise. They will be able to advise you on a safe routine should you wish to continue exercising while pregnant.

– If you have an injury that is giving you pain, you should consult a Pilates teacher before you undertake any exercise. Sometimes it is better to rest the injury than to start work on it immediately. This general advice is given by Pilates teachers, physiotherapists and other bodywork practitioners.

– Similarly, if you are taking strong painkillers you are advised to wait until the pain has eased sufficiently for you to stop taking them. The reason for this is that painkillers mask the pain, and while you exercise you will be unaware of any extra pain being caused by your movements, possibly leading to further damage. There is a saying 'no pain, no gain'. People commonly believe that they must force themselves through the pain while exercising in order for it to be doing them good, but the opposite is true. Your muscles should definitely not be pushed to the point of pain. Pain should not be confused with feeling the muscle contract as you exercise it, especially when you are beginning an exercise programme. That is why you should not push your body beyond its limits – only go as far in an exercise as is comfortable.

– Do not exercise after eating a heavy meal as you may experience severe cramping pains.

– Similarly, do not exercise after drinking alcohol as, apart from anything else, you will not be in the right frame of mind to concentrate.

– If you are undergoing medical treatment, consult your medical practitioner before embarking on any new form of exercise. Also, remember to tell your Pilates teacher about any specific ailments or injuries from which you suffer.

The second-century Roman emperor and philosopher Marcus Aurelius wrote, **'The body ought to be stable and free from all irregularity, whether in rest or in motion.'** This ideal is difficult to achieve in the contemporary world. We now expect to gain maximum results from all aspects of our lives, yet we rarely have enough time to examine the efficacy of our efforts. Whether we are working or relaxing, our bodies seem to be in a constant state of unease.

Many adults are required to sit for long periods at work, often at computers. But sitting for extended periods is an unnatural activity. If, for example, you observe children (see pictures), you will notice how they hate to sit for any length of time, preferring instead to roam and roll about, until they are forced into sitting for a class at school, or when they must do so as evidence of good behaviour. Very often, we learn our postural habits, whether good or bad, while we are still young.

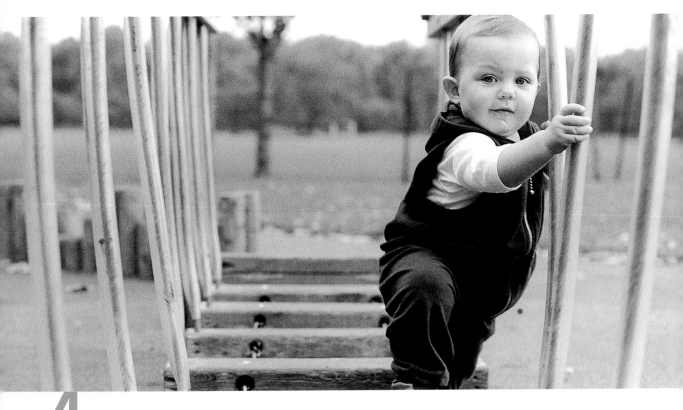

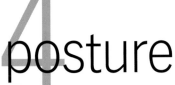

4 posture

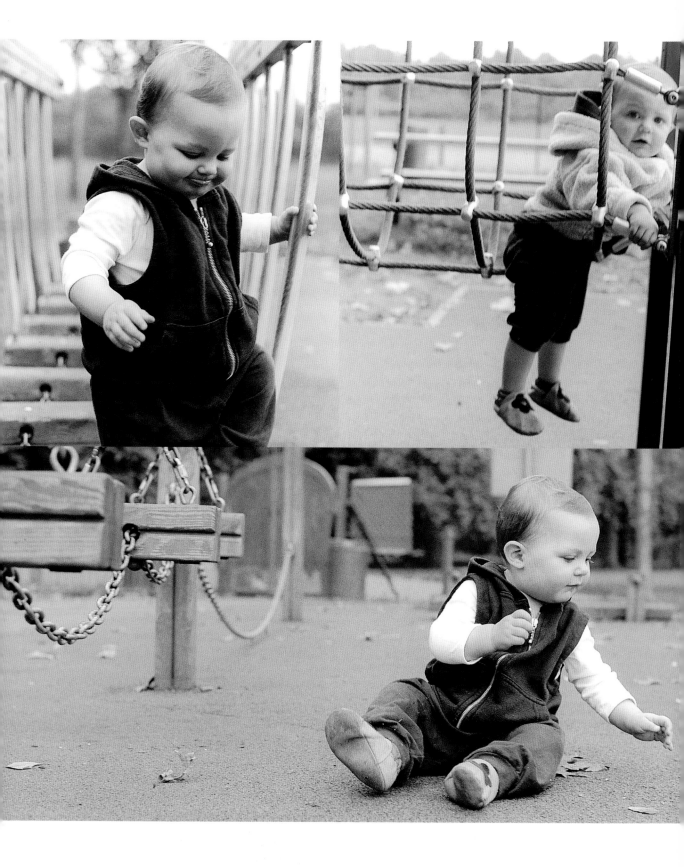

Good posture

We are often told that we need to improve our posture, yet most of us are uncertain about what good posture really is. The Victorians valued the straight back so much that young ladies were trained to have one by wearing a back board. This perception of good posture lingered on into the second half of this century, and it is only with the growing interest in Pilates, the Alexander Technique and the Feldenkrais Method that we are learning that good posture is about a lot more than a straight back.

Good posture lends balance to the limbs, allowing movements, such as walking, to be performed smoothly. Everyone has their own unique way of walking, so conforming to a single ideal is simply not practical, but an awareness of your body's posture can add synergy and control to an otherwise unconscious movement.

Observing the way people walk often provides an insight into their personality and their emotions. These appear to interact with the muscles that facilitate the walking movement and those in the upper body so as to create a personal style. Over time this posture becomes the norm for that person. They will be unaware of the tension held in the muscles, which is constantly pulling and twisting the skeleton, as well as tightening the muscles. They are also unaware that this incorrect use of muscles and joints is uneconomical, leading to a waste of energy and fatigue.

Nowadays, most people do very little walking, which makes the way we sit more important. How do we approach sitting down? Usually without much thought. As we sit down we tend to slouch and compress the spine so that it curves round unnaturally and shortens the muscles. Over time, these shortened muscles resist the attempt to lengthen them, and this brings discomfort. By re-educating the body by doing the Pilates Core Stabilization exercises, you can adopt a good sitting posture more comfortably.

But sitting at work and in the home is only part of the problem, and the solution, of poor sitting posture. Awareness of muscle and skeletal function and their re-education are the only lasting solution to posture problems and the difficulties that result from them. For example, we should be aware of the way that the back works to withstand the different strains placed on it. The three natural curves of the spine – two hollows and

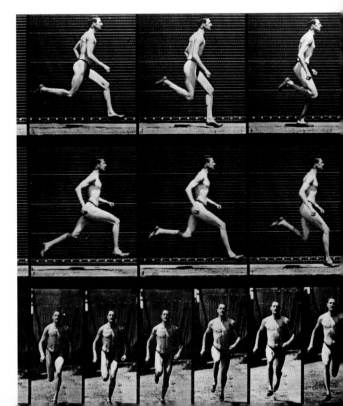

posture

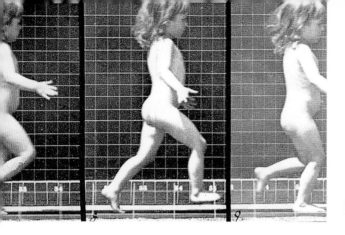

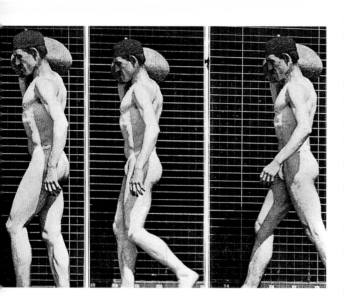

Postural problems

The posture of the foetus in the womb is our starting point in life. If you look at a picture of an embryo you will see that the spinal column is curved like a letter 'C'. Once free of the confines of the womb, the baby's spine gradually elongates, and at this point two new curves develop in the spine, forming two hollows. The first is at the neck and is called the cervical curve. This forms so that we can hold our heads up. When the baby learns to crawl, and eventually to walk, another hollow appears in the lower back, and this is called the lumbar curve. The third curve in the spine is a convex curve called the thoracic curve. There are many problems that can arise with the spine, but kyphosis, lordosis and scoliosis are the most commonly seen spinal deformities. In some cases the tendency is genetic, while in others it is caused by unbalanced posture. These conditions, which are quite common, can be rectified by using Pilates exercises.

Kyphosis

The kyphosis is situated between the shoulder blades and is the only part of the spine that has kept its convex shape. The kyphosis is normal, but an increase in it is defined as abnormal – this is what is commonly called a round back. True abnormal kyphosis may be confused with round shoulders, which is when the back is hunched from side to side, rather than a hunch being created from front to back. Often seen in adolescents when they adopt a slouching posture, this is known as 'postural kyphosis' and is not a real spinal deformity at

one hump – help it to withstand greater force than if it were perfectly straight. A normal lower-back curve supports the anatomy of the lower back and prevents injury. These natural curves have the same function as a shock absorber. If the spine were completely straight, it would be extremely vulnerable to shock.

The spine is made up of bony vertebrae, cushioned by discs. The discs consist of a jelly-like centre (nucleus) surrounded by a fibrous ring-like structure (annulus). Surrounding the vertebrae and discs are muscles and ligaments that provide movement and stability. Poor posture – for example, sitting hunched over your desk or slumping on the sofa – can cause the nucleus to push against the fibrous annulus and cause pain.

all. Kyphosis can sometimes be associated with osteoporosis, and is therefore frequently seen in post-menopausal women.

Conventional treatment for increased kyphosis is physiotherapy, and it is rare that surgery is recommended. The tendency to form an abnormal kyphosis may be inherited. Families with a history of spinal abnormalities are advised to have their children examined regularly so that they can start a preventive exercise programme at as early an age as possible.

Scoliosis

Scoliosis is a lateral or sideways curvature of the spine, with a rotation of the spine often involved as well. There is a tendency for scoliosis to be genetically inherited, and for it to be more common in females. When it is not genetic, functional scoliosis can be caused by repeated actions, such as carrying a shoulder bag. In the majority of cases, however, the cause is unknown. This is called 'idiopathic scoliosis', and it generally first appears in childhood or in adolescence.

A severe scoliosis can affect the position of the ribs, and may disturb the natural placement of internal organs. In such cases, the person's appearance and their general health are affected. The kind of health risks that might arise from a severe scoliosis include neurological problems from pressure on the nerves, and lung problems. A lateral curve that occurs in the lower spine may also affect the upper spine as the person compensates for the curve in their lower back.

Lordosis

A degree of curvature in the lower back is quite normal, but if there is an excessive hollowing in the area of the lumbar spine then the condition is defined as lordosis. This inward curvature of the spine tends to make the stomach appear more prominent than it really is, causing the person to look overweight when in fact they are not. In some people the curve is flexible.

Each of these postural problems can be helped by using Pilates exercises, especially if an experienced teacher creates a tailor-made exercise programme, and monitors the person's progress while ensuring that they do not try to work beyond their limits. For example, with Pilates exercises many people have found that they have been able to ease their scoliosis, which can be the most problematic of the spinal abnormalities. This, of course, does not happen in days or weeks, but will take place with regular practice over several years.

posture

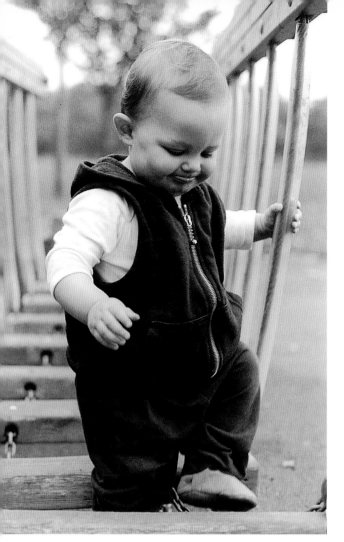

balance and ease. It is this unease that tires us and sends us looking for somewhere to sit down.

Pilates teaches a way to stand that allows us to rest in the position with our muscles relaxed and our balance centred. It will probably take some practice before it becomes second nature, but once it is achieved it will mean you tire less easily, feel taller and are more relaxed in your environment.

How to stand

1. Stand with your feet hip-width apart.
2. Make sure that both your legs are facing forward.
3. Your legs should be straight but the knees should not be locked back into the joint.
4. Allow your arms to rest naturally at your sides, falling over the middle of your hips.
5. Feel your weight being supported by the middle of each foot.
6. Do not rock back, allowing the heels to take your weight, or place your weight on the balls of your feet.

Standing

Standing is an activity that many people frequently find uncomfortable. Often when we stand still we do not know what to do with our bodies. We put our weight on one leg, bending the other, then we shift our weight to the other leg. We attempt to stand up straight, but we lock our knees and push the pelvis forward, creating an exaggerated hollow in the lower spine. At the same time, we do not know what to do with our arms. We fold them across the front of our body, clasp our hands behind our backs or place our hands on our hips. It is as if we have no sense of the centre of gravity within the body, but if we can find it, it will hold us in a position of

Sitting

Like standing, sitting is something we often don't do very well. We sit balanced on one hip bone, then we shift to the other. We cross our legs or sit with one leg underneath us. We wriggle around in our seats, trying to find a position that will feel comfortable. When we eventually do find a comfortable position, it does not last long. We try to find external solutions to this, such as lumbar supports on chairs or car seats. The trouble with these, though, is that they are not suitable for most people. They are too low down to give support where it is needed. Instead they tend to push the lumbar spine forward, and this in turn pushes the abdominal muscles and the internal organs forward.

When looking for a chair that will properly support your back and allow you to adopt good sitting posture, you should check for the following:

1. You should be able to sit comfortably with your whole thigh supported by the seat of the chair.
2. You should be able to place both of your feet flat on the floor.
3. The back support should be as high as your shoulder blades. The backs of many office chairs are either lower or higher than this.

Remember to sit with your weight evenly distributed, your knees should be slightly apart in order to support the weight, and your feet should be together, underneath the knees.

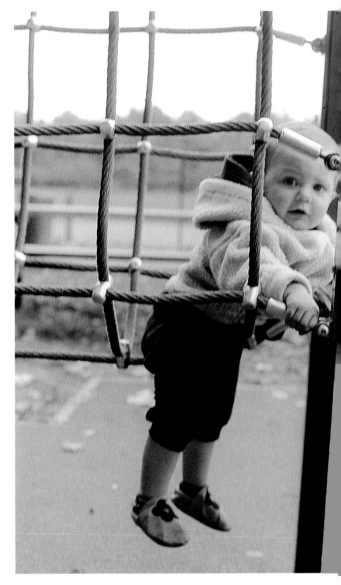

posture

Lying

We spend approximately one-third of each day lying down. Again we do not give much thought to this, we just do it, and as we are sleeping for most of this time, we are unaware of our position. Lying down should be our ultimate position of rest, but still we manage to contort ourselves in various ways that put strain on our muscles and limit our blood circulation.

Sleeping positions

Many people sleep on their stomachs. This is not a good position as it does not support the spine. Also, when people sleep in this position they usually bend one leg up, which twists the spine. To breathe properly while lying on the stomach, the head has to be turned to one side. This not only twists the neck but can also trap nerves in the neck, leading to a feeling of numbness or 'pins and needles' during sleep or on waking. It can also create functional scoliosis (see page 34).

The best positions for sleeping in are on the back or the sides. If you have a lower-back problem it can be helpful to sleep with pillows between your knees. This is also recommended if you are pregnant, when it can be extremely difficult to find a comfortable sleeping position and you are more likely to suffer with circulation problems. Similarly, if you have a lordosis (see page 34), pillows placed under the thighs or buttocks can provide more comfort while sleeping. Many people claim that they find it impossible to sleep with pillows between or under their legs, but it usually takes only a short time before they appreciate the benefits and forget that the pillows are even there.

Beds and pillows

Hard mattresses are not good. Rather, it is better to have a firm mattress that has some give in it, allowing some moulding to the body contours. The number of pillows you use depends on the density of the pillows, but one or two is the norm. If the pillow is of a higher density, one should be sufficient for most people. It is important that the neck is fully supported by the pillow, and that there are no gaps between the neck and the pillow to put extra strain on the neck muscles.

In the first stage of learning Pilates, you listen to the teacher and then follow their instructions. For a while you continue to practise exactly what you have been taught. In time you come to the second stage, which is when you believe you have learned your lessons so well that you can now start to improve upon them with your own ideas. Experimentation is a necessary part of the evolution of theory and practice, but it is effective only when the fundamental concept is completely understood.

When you learn, you interpret what you are told in a particular way. You programme that information into your mind and it is set there. Your interpretation will probably be subtly different from what you have been shown. You then need to be reminded of the original method by the teacher, because it is only correct practice that gives a good result.

Remember, always return to the basics before you move on.

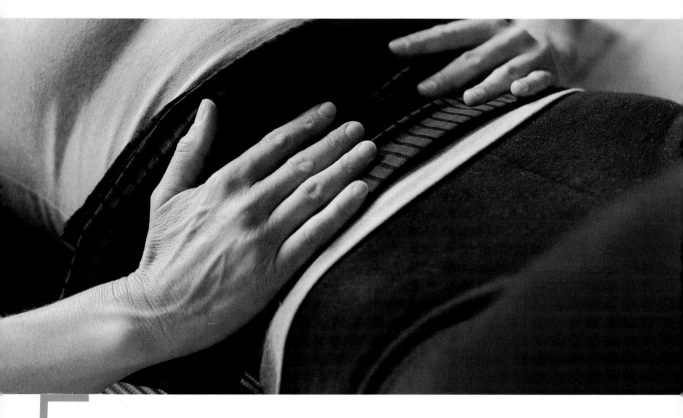

5 core stabilization

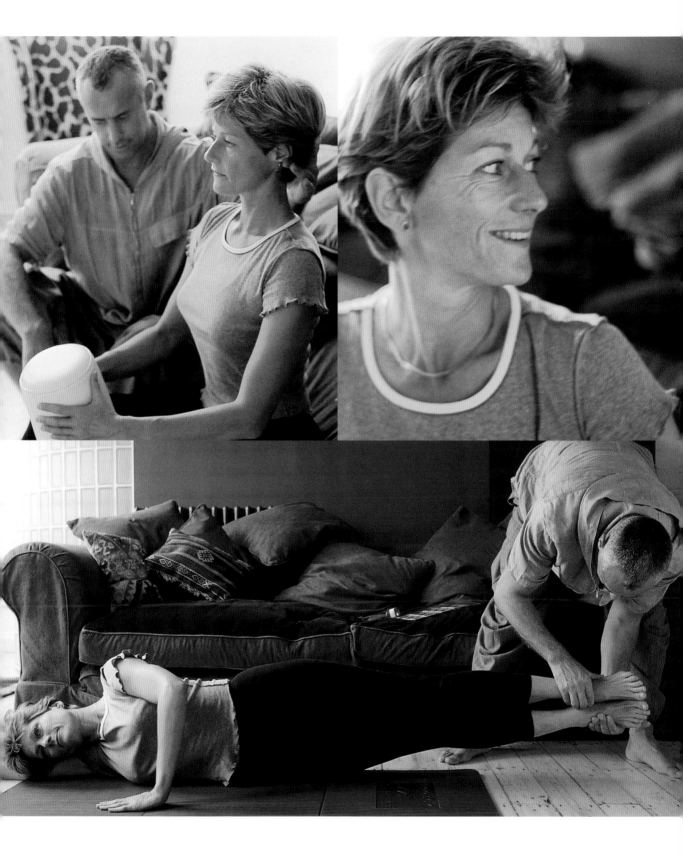

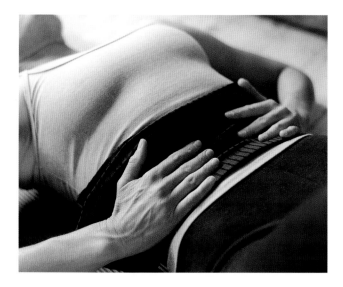

Core stabilization

Core Stabilization is the focal point of Pilates. It could be described as balancing the centre, or building a strong centre by beginning with strengthening the internal muscles. Essentially, it means creating a circle of strength around the centre of the trunk, as the muscles at the centre of the body are fundamental to the health of the whole. Strengthening the muscles in this area protects the spine and the internal organs. It also gives you the ability to control the upper and lower body areas from the core while still protecting and stabilizing the spine.

Core Stabilization is also a set of exercises that provide the basics of the Pilates technique. It is to the exact performance of these exercises that the student must always return. The set of 17 exercises provided here works the key muscles necessary for good posture, which in turn has an effect on the rest of the body and the mind.

Recovery from most injuries and management of most muscular conditions can be aided by using the Core Stabilization exercises. They strengthen and lengthen the muscles and, in the process, free the whole body. This holistic approach to treating injuries and musculoskeletal conditions makes Pilates a method, not just a random collection of exercises.

Each person would be assessed by the Pilates teacher according to their individual problem. Muscles and joints do not work in isolation but rather in synergy. This is called musculo-skeletal harmonization. For example, if a person comes to a Pilates studio with a knee problem, the teacher will not just look at how that knee is functioning; they will also assess the functioning of the muscles and joints of the whole leg and the core muscles that support the whole spine. The reason for this is that in some cases pain in the knee is the result of dysfunction in the lower back, and it is this 'referred pain' that travels through the nerves. In this case it would be wrong to exercise only the knee when the problem originates in the lower back. Also, after an injury the body adjusts and compensates by altering the body's natural alignment and balance. The Core Stabilization exercises help to restore natural alignment and posture. Finally, they also allow stabilization of the central postural muscles of the body, making it ready for work on the upper and lower parts. In all the exercises, the stabilization of the lumbar spine, or lower back, is key. The exercises aim to strengthen the muscles which support this area, creating a firm abdomen to protect and support the lower back. In achieving this, the role of the pelvic floor cannot be emphasized too strongly.

core stabilization

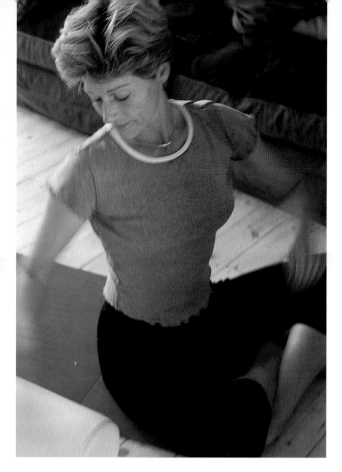

In Pilates, pelvic floor exercises have a slightly different function. They are critical to creating internal Core Stabilization, which then supports the work on the external skeletal muscles. Control of the pelvic floor while breathing correctly is the starting point for all the exercises in this book. Therefore it is worth taking time to learn them properly before moving on. The more familiar you are with them, the more you will be able to focus on the exercises that follow.

The pelvic floor and wall are like an internal cylinder made of muscle. It is a group of internal muscles that are located just inside the pelvic cavity. Their strength or weakness affects the functioning of not just the pelvic area, but also the legs and ultimately the upper body. Strong pelvic floor muscles help to resist the pull of gravity and so stop the abdominal organs pressing on those below. Strengthening this area is important for both men and women, although women may experience more obvious benefits as the pelvic floor is

weakened by childbirth. You will know that you are using them if, on tightening the pelvic muscles, you feel them trembling inside; your whole body will also feel as though it is lifting.

Practising core stabilization exercises

Mindfulness, or concentration, when exercising is an essential part of Pilates, and differentiates it from conventional exercise. This may take some time to achieve. If you practise meditation you will probably be familiar with the instruction to bring the mind back to the breath when your 'mind chatter' interrupts your concentration. When practising Pilates exercises, particularly at the beginning, you must focus your attention on what each part of your body is doing, and feeling, during the exercise. This is obvious when you consider that all movement starts with a message from the brain. If you focus well you will soon become aware of when your body is at ease and when it is not. Your ability to concentrate will increase as you become automatically aware of any incorrect movements.

You will also need to learn how to exercise in a relaxed manner. The term relaxation has a very precise meaning in Pilates; it means without undue tension rather than allowing the body to flop. The way to achieve this is to focus on the part of the body you are about to exercise and adjust yourself so that your body is in the correct position to begin the exercise. Preparing yourself for an exercise, rather than just going straight into it, enables you to release muscle tension before you begin, making the exercise much more efficient. You will also need

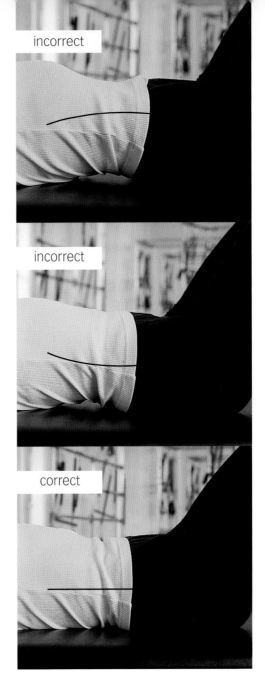

incorrect

incorrect

correct

to think about the coordination of your movements. As with all exercises, there is a lot to think about, especially if you are trying to follow instructions from a book.

One solution is to record the steps of each of the Core Stabilization exercises onto a tape. The more good practice you do and the more familiar you become with the exercises, the better your coordination will be.

This may sound a little difficult but it will come with practice. Remember, most Pilates exercises should be performed slowly and with flowing movements. The latter will increase your ability to control the correct muscles and reduce tension as your body becomes familiar with the sequence of movements. If you take all the exercises slowly to begin with, it will be easier for you to combine the elements of concentration, relaxation and coordination.

Neutral spine

While practising Pilates exercises you will be working in what Pilates teachers call 'neutral spine'. Essentially this means maintaining the natural curve of your back during exercise. To find out if you are doing this, lie down on the floor with your knees bent. If you tilt your pelvis up, you will lose the natural curve in your back as it is pressed into the floor. If you tilt your pelvis down, your lower back becomes over-arched. The neutral position of the spine is when the pelvis is balanced so that the curve in the lower spine is not lost by pressing your back onto the floor or when your back is over-arched, leaving a gap between your back and the floor. You will need to take some time to work with this to get it right for you, as everybody is different.

Before you begin the exercises there are two other key elements of Pilates that need to be learned: correct breathing and the role of the pelvic floor.

core stabilization

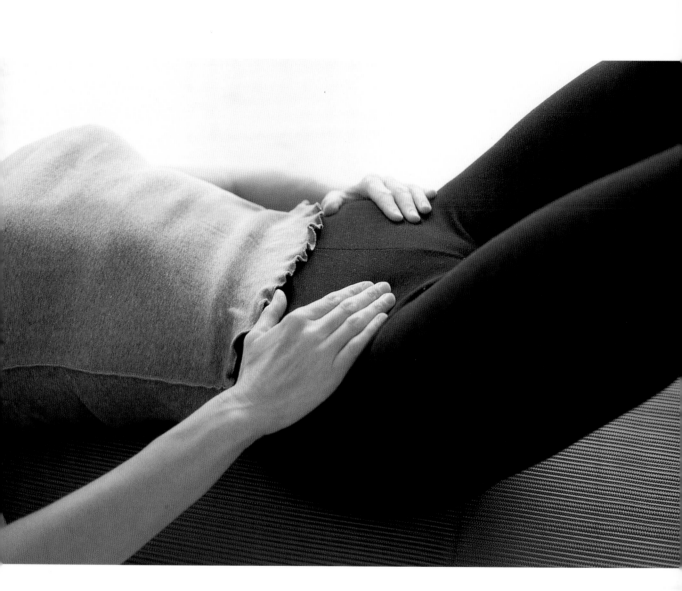

Correct breathing

When we inhale, oxygen is drawn into the lungs and from there it enters the blood stream and is carried around the body. Anything that impedes the amount or quality of oxygen being inhaled reduces the amount of oxygen entering the blood, and as a result impairs the health of all our cells. Increasing your oxygen supply will make you more tranquil, and will improve brain function, blood circulation and physical coordination. For these reasons breathing is central to Pilates, since it focuses on relaxation, and mind and body coordination.

There are many factors in modern life that work against our ability to increase our oxygen supply. One of the major factors is air pollution. When the air quality is poor, so is the quality of the oxygen we inhale. Poor air is also deficient in negative ions, which are known to improve physical and mental health. The other main factors are lifestyle habits, such as smoking, excessive sitting and prolonged stress. People are generally aware that smoking damages breathing, but they tend to be less aware that poor posture and stress also contribute to poor breathing habits that may result in overall poor health.

Breathing is one of the few body functions that is both automatic and voluntary. Most of us will take millions of breaths in our lifetime without giving it a thought, yet we have the ability to control our breathing; if we start to breathe too rapidly, we can learn how to slow it down. The way we breathe affects our health and our emotions. Most of us use only the upper part of our lungs when we breathe, and we tend to take shallow breaths that do not provide us with enough oxygen. We also breathe in a way that makes us expand only our chest and raise our shoulders. This common way of breathing uses the wrong muscles. It ignores the diaphragm muscle, which expands and contracts the ribs to allow oxygen to entirely fill both lungs, not just a part of them.

Breathing away stress

If you are in a state of fear or panic it is likely that someone will tell you to take a deep breath. Controlling your breathing is one way of controlling the symptoms of stress. Meditation, yoga and a number of stress-management techniques, such as autogenic training, as well as Pilates, all focus on conscious breathing. When you are feeling stressed, your body will send a surge of adrenalin through the sympathetic nervous system causing your breathing, as well as your heart rate, to change. Breathing becomes faster and shallower, and consequently you do not take in enough oxygen. To compensate for this you breathe even faster to try and take in more oxygen. In some cases this cycle results in hyperventilation, which in turn causes dizziness or fainting.

Eastern breathing techniques

Breathing technique is emphasized in practices such as yoga and chi kung. In these, the student breathes deeply from the diaphragm, expanding the abdomen on the 'in' breath, and thus slowing down the rate of breathing. When people begin classes they are asked to time the number of exhalations they make in a minute. The usual number is around 13–15 with unregulated breathing. When you practise deep breathing, this measurement will drop to three or four exhalations per minute. Chi kung and yoga masters can bring it down to one. However, the breathing technique used in Pilates is very different from this.

The Pilates breathing technique

Pilates teaches lateral breathing. This is a type of breathing in which you avoid expanding the abdomen. The aim is to use the thoracic and back muscles to expand the ribcage sideways, and make room for the lungs to expand. The reason for not extending the abdomen with air is that when the lower abdominal muscle is stretched, the lower back is left unsupported and therefore unprotected.

Pilates breathing helps to improve not only your breathing but also your physical and mental health. It also functions as an integral part of each exercise. Following the breathing instructions given with each exercise will allow you to gain the maximum results from your practise. Remember that in Pilates the emphasis is placed on the 'out' breath.

core stabilization

Pilates breathing exercises

Before you begin, practise breathing in through the nose and out through the mouth. If you are unused to this, you will find it easier to try it out before following the breathing instructions. Remember that when you are breathing while performing an exercise, the movement must be performed on the 'out' breath. The reason for this is that the diaphragm lifts as you breathe out, causing the stomach muscles to pull in tightly, and the spine to lengthen. This creates a strong centre, which is fundamental to the Core Stabilization process. Finally, do not relax your stomach muscles on the 'in' breath while performing an exercise, as this can cause you to lose correct postural alignment, and to use the wrong muscles.

Even if you have problems coordinating the breathing exercise with other elements of Pilates exercises, never hold your breath, no matter what. It is better to breathe in a natural way than hold the breath, which puts some pressure on the lungs and heart.

aim

To coordinate your breathing with your muscle control.

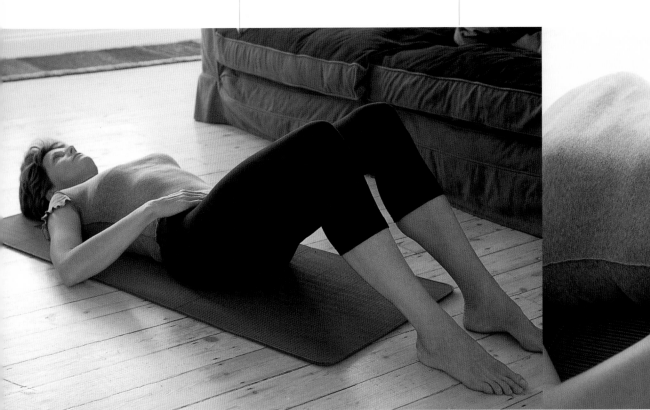

preparation

Begin by lying down on your exercise mat.

Keep your feet hip-width apart and your knees bent.

Now place your hands on your abdomen between the hip bones, fingertips touching.

Do not apply pressure with your hands, simply allow them to rest there.

Breathe in through your nose.

1 breathing

2

3

watchpoint

– Do not allow the spine or pelvis to move. The same applies to the Pelvic Floor exercise (see pages 48–49).

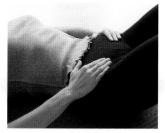

Begin in the same starting position as for the Breathing exercise.

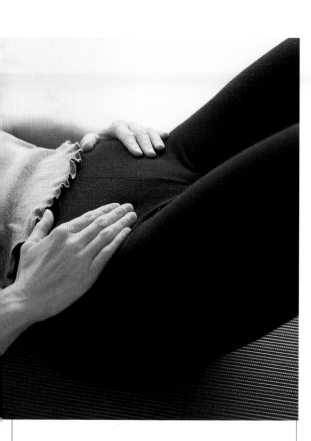

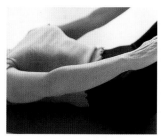

Raise your hands and arms to the height of your knees, keeping your arms straight.

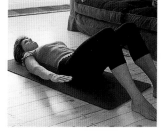

As you do this lower your hands and arms towards the floor, and visualize that they are trying to press a float down through the water, thus creating a feeling of resistance. End with your hands on the floor.

Repeat 6–10 times.

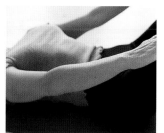

Breathe in through your nose. On the **'out' breath**, feel the abdominal muscles pulling in towards the spine.

On the **'out' breath**, feel your abdominal muscles fall into the pelvic cavity.

As this occurs, consciously take it further and pull the abdominal muscles in towards the spine.

Repeat 6–10 times.

4

variation

aim

To work the pelvic floor muscles progressively deeper.

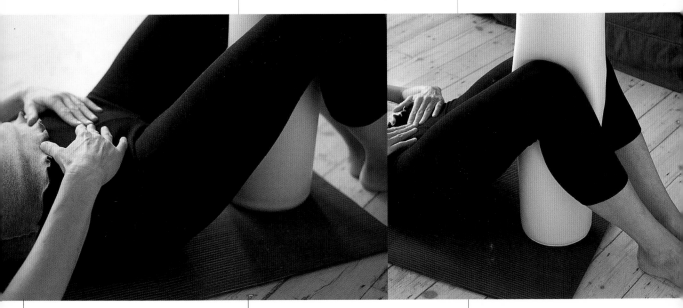

preparation

Begin by lying down with your feet together and your knees bent.

Put your hands on your abdomen and place the cushion between your knees.

Take a small breath through your nose.

Breathing out, in sequence, tighten and pull up the pelvic floor, squeeze your buttocks gently and squeeze the cushion between your knees.

Hold this position for **3–6 breaths**.

If you feel that 3 breaths is too long, squeeze on the **'out' breath** and release on the **'in' breath**.

Repeat 6–10 times.

1 pelvic floor

2

3

watchpoint
– Do not allow the spine or pelvis to move, this will ensure that you maintain a neutral spine position.

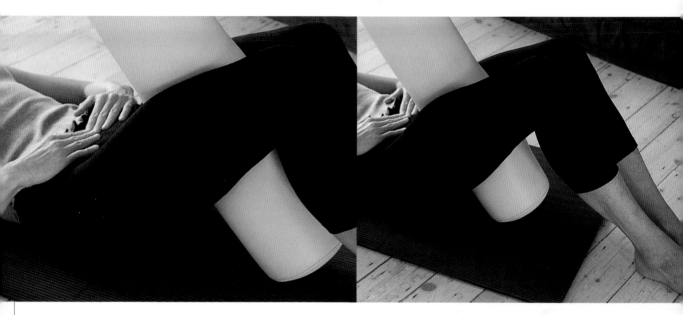

Move the cushion halfway up the inner thighs, **take a small breath** through your nose and then **repeat** steps 2 and 3.

Move the cushion to between the upper thighs, **take a small breath** through your nose and then **repeat** steps 2 and 3.

Moving the position of the cushion changes the way that you use the pelvic floor muscles. When you place the cushion between the upper thighs you will really feel the lower abdominal muscles working hard.

variation

aim

– To strengthen the lower abdominal and mobilize the lower back.

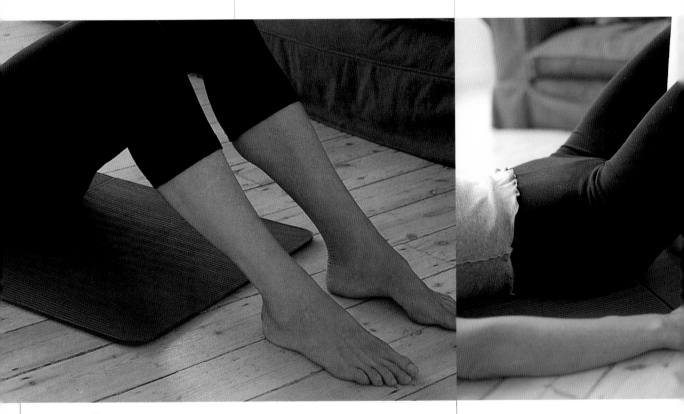

preparation

Begin by lying on the floor with your knees bent. Your feet and knees should be hip-width apart.

Your arms should rest beside you, with the palms of your hands flat on the floor.

Breathe in through your nose. Pull up your pelvic floor and pull in your lower stomach muscles.

Place a cushion between your thighs, just above your knees.

Gently squeeze the cushion between your legs, although not as hard as for the Pelvic Floor exercise (see pages 48–49).

1 pelvic tilt

2

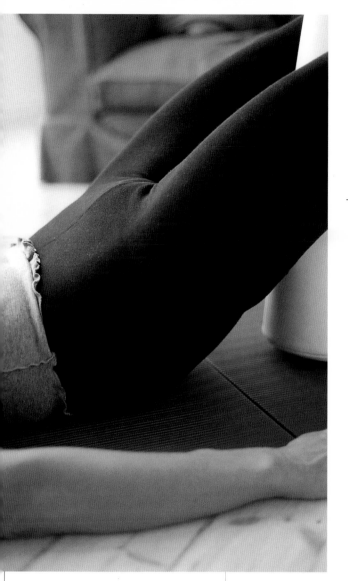

watchpoint

– The aim of this exercise is to use your muscles rather than your joints.

Breathing out, tilt the pelvis up, rising one vertebra at a time, until the lumbar spine is flat on the floor.

Stay still, holding your pelvic floor and abdominals.

Take a small breath in.

Breathing out, slowly lower your spine down to the neutral spine position while still holding your pelvic floor and abdominal muscles.

Repeat 6–10 times.

3

4

5

aim

– To strengthen the abdominal muscles and hamstrings, and mobilize the thoracic and lumbar spine.

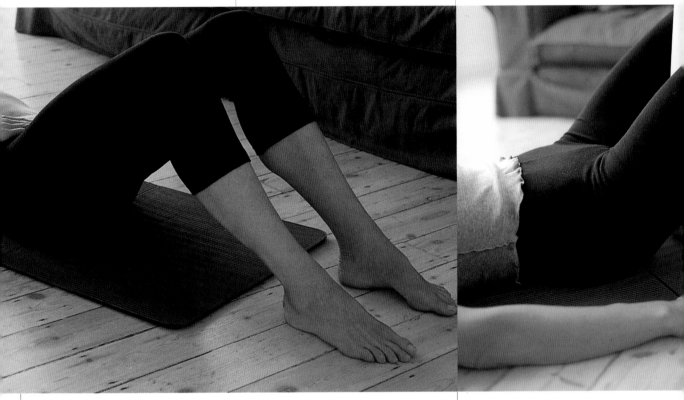

preparation

Begin by lying on the floor with your knees bent. Your feet and knees should be hip-width apart.

Your arms should rest beside you, with the palms of your hands flat on the floor.

Breathe in, pull up your pelvic floor and pull in your lower stomach muscles.

Place a cushion between your thighs, just above your knees.

Gently squeeze the cushion between your legs

1 pelvic lift

2

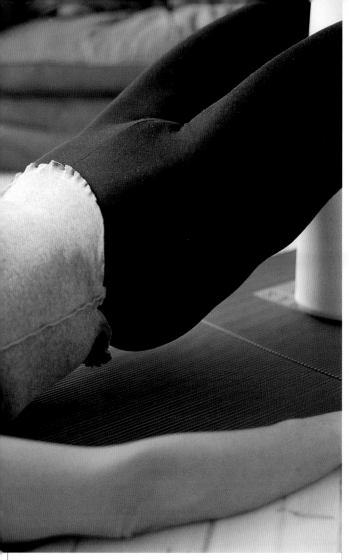

watchpoints

– Do not arch your lumbar spine or allow your knees to fall any further apart – consciously think of lengthening the curves.

– When raising and lowering your spine, always aim to peel the spine off the mat – imagine removing a plaster slowly.

– Bring your tailbone down onto the mat last. Do not allow it to touch the mat before the rest of your spine does.

– Keep your pelvic floor and stomach muscles working; do not let them go until you have finished your repetitions.

Breathing out, tilt your pelvis up, peeling each vertebra from the floor one at a time.

You will now be resting on your thoracic vertebrae, just below the shoulder blades.

While holding this position, **breathe in** again.

Breathing out, lower your spine slowly back down to the floor, again taking care to lower one vertebra at a time.

Repeat 6–10 times.

3

4

aim

– To lengthen and strengthen the internal and external oblique muscles.

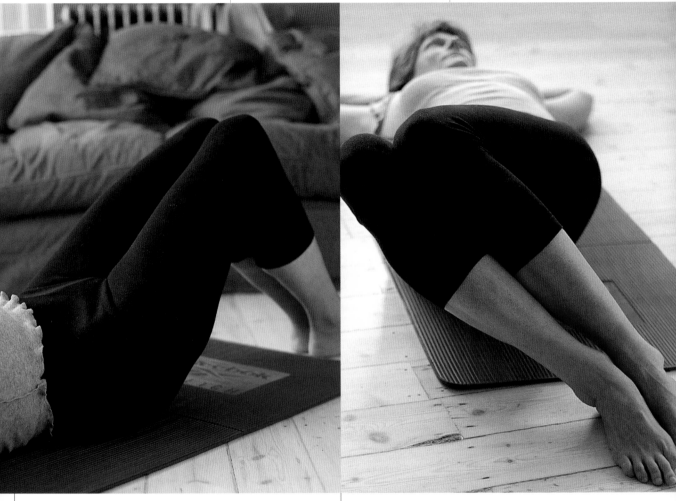

preparation

Begin by lying down with your knees and feet together and your knees raised.

Place your hands behind your head with your elbows pointing out to the sides.

Breathe in, pull up your pelvic floor and pull in your stomach muscles.

Breathing out, bring your legs halfway towards one side.

Once there, hold the position and **breathe in**.

Breathe out and bring your legs back to the middle.

1

2

small hip roll

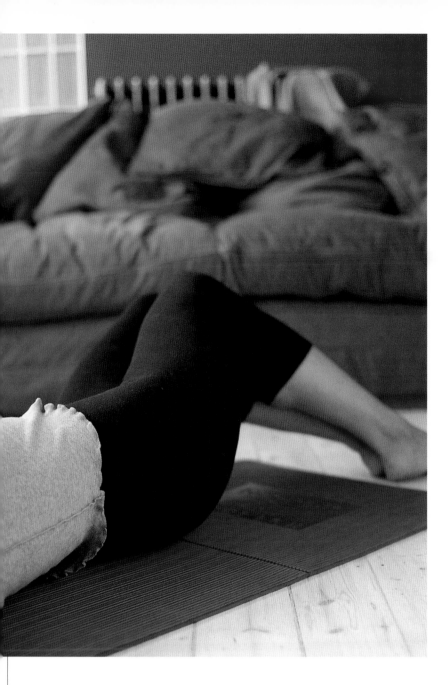

Repeat the movement to your other side.

Repeat 3–6 times each side.

watchpoints

– This exercises your stomach muscles, so remember to tighten your oblique abdominals when breathing out.
– Do not try to push your legs over too far towards the floor.

3

aim

– To strengthen the abdominal muscles, and stretch the hip flexors and lower back.

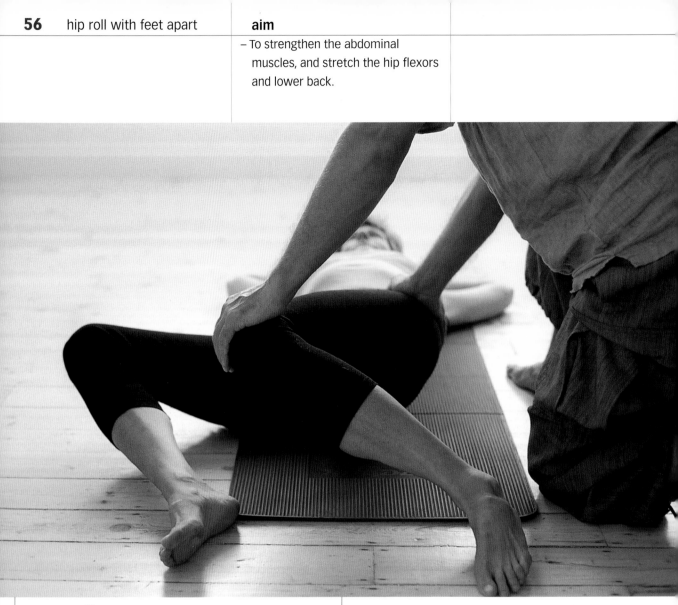

preparation

Begin by lying down with your knees and feet slightly wider than hip-width apart, keeping them parallel.

Place your hands behind your head with your elbows pointing out to the sides.

Breathe in, pull up your pelvic floor and pull in your lower stomach muscles.

Breathing out, bring your legs over to one side. The soles of your feet will come off the floor when you do this. Very gently push as far over to the side as possible without lifting your back off the mat.

Hold the position and **breathe in**.

1 hip roll with feet apart 2

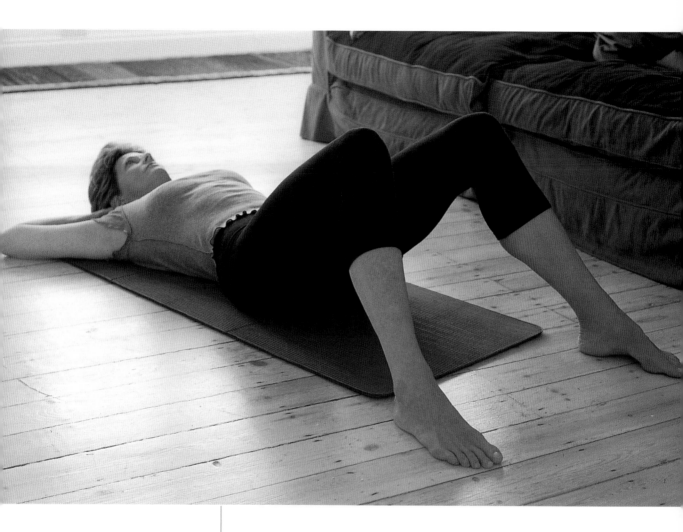

Breathing out, pull your legs back to the centre, using your abdominal muscles to do the pulling.

Repeat the movement to the other side.

Repeat 3–6 times each side.

3

4

watchpoint

– Imagine a cord attached to your navel, pulling your spine towards the floor, or a hand on your hip, pushing you down.

aim

- To strengthen the deep interior waist muscle – the Quadratus lumborum – and the transverse and oblique abdominals.

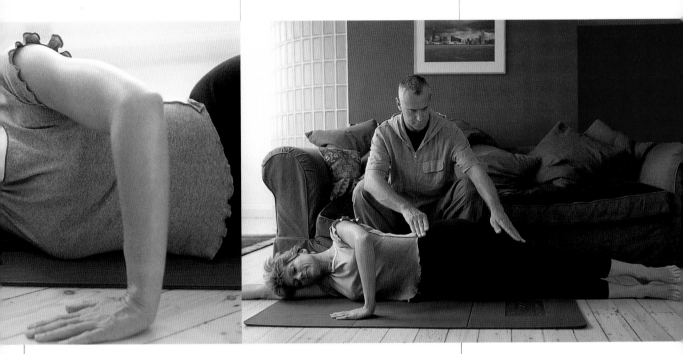

preparation

Lie on one side, ensuring that your body is in a straight line. Your ear, the middle of your shoulder, and your hip and ankle should all be aligned. Check that your feet are pointing down, not flexed forward.

The arm of the side on which you are lying should be raised above your head, palm facing up. Rest your head on your arm. Place your other arm in front of you, with the palm of your hand on the floor.

Once in position, make sure that both your shoulders and your neck are relaxed. Stretch both your legs away from the waist, making the waist long.

Pull·up the pelvic floor and pull the stomach muscles in towards the spine.

Now **breathe in**.

Breathing out, lift both legs about 10cm (4in) from the floor.

As you do this, imagine that your ankles are bound together.

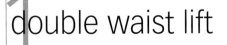

1 double waist lift

2

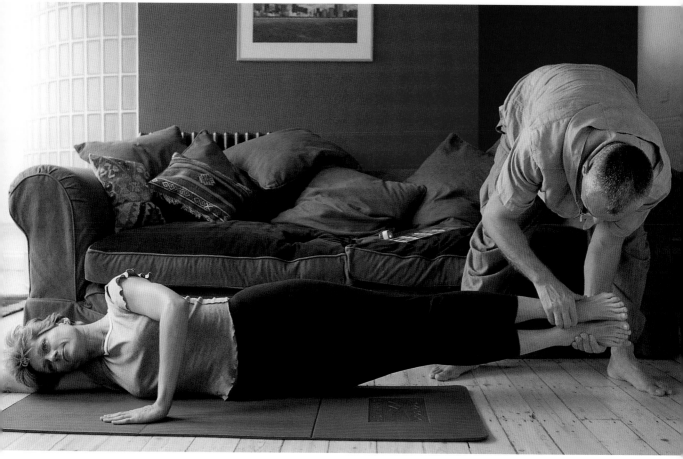

Breathe in and slowly lower
your legs to the floor.

Repeat 6–10 times each side.

3

watchpoints
– Beware of arching your lower back and twisting your
pelvis or shoulders.
– Do not shorten your waist.
– Do not let go of your pelvic floor.

aim

– To strengthen the lats, the Quadratus lumborum, and the transverse and oblique abdominals.

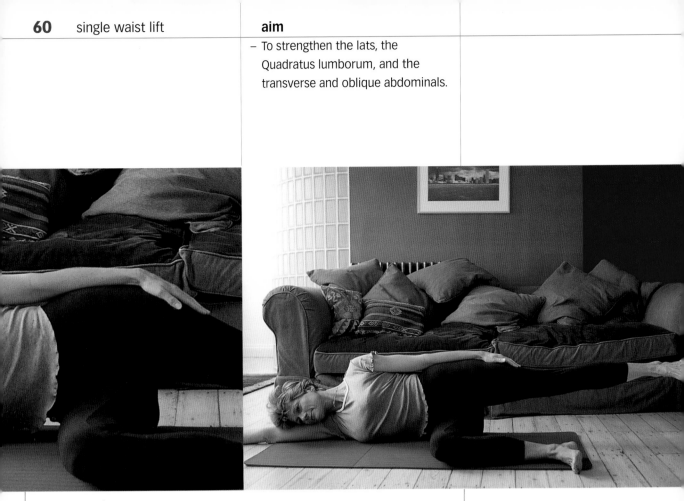

preparation

Begin in the same starting position as in the Double Waist Lift (see page 58), but instead of having your upper arm in front of your body, allow it to rest on your side with your hand on your thigh.

Bend the leg nearest to the floor in front of you and flex your feet.

Once in the position, pull your shoulders down towards your hip and stretch your fingers towards your knee.

Lengthen your waist by pushing your heel downwards slightly.

Breathe in, pulling up your pelvic floor, pulling in your lower stomach muscles and tightening your waist and buttock muscles.

Breathing out, lift your leg up to hip height.

As you do this, reach with your fingers towards your knee.

1 single waist lift

2

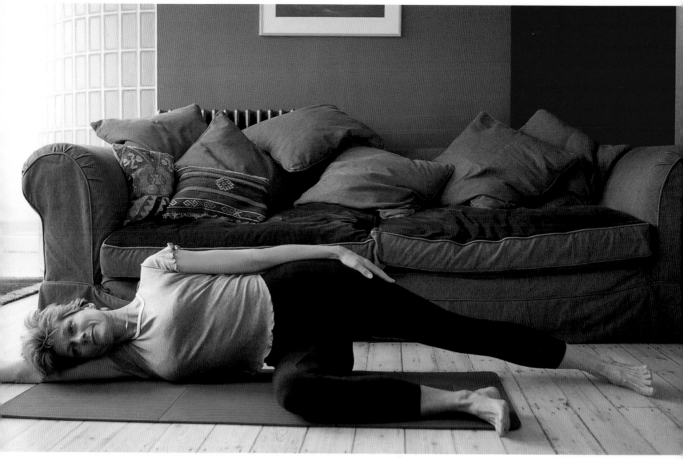

Breathe in and bring your leg down, pulling the pelvic floor up and the stomach muscles in as you do so.

Repeat 6–10 times each side.

3

watchpoint
– Do not arch your lower back or move out of alignment.

aim

– To mobilize the thoracic spine and lengthen the abdominal muscles.

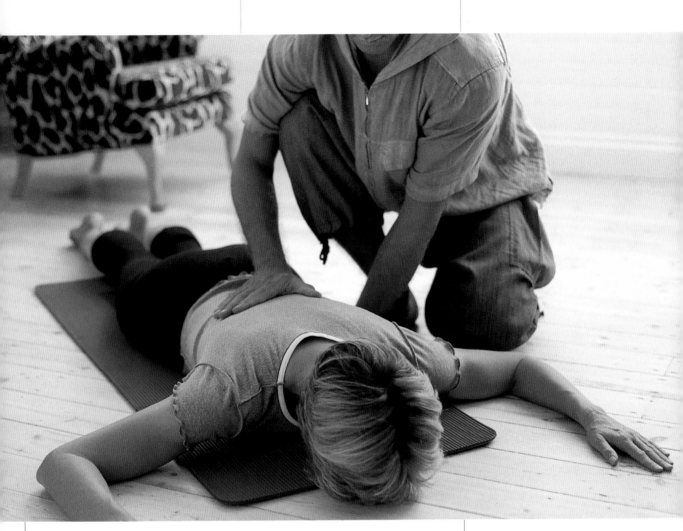

preparation

Begin by lying on your stomach. You can rest your forehead on a folded towel if you like.

Place your hands above your head, with your palms facing down and your fingertips pointing straight ahead. Make sure that your elbows are stretched out to the side at shoulder level.

Breathe in, pull up your pelvic floor and pull in your stomach muscles.

Breathing out, peel your chest up from the floor, ensuring that your elbows remain on the floor.

Hold the position and **breathe in**.

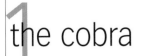

the cobra

1

2

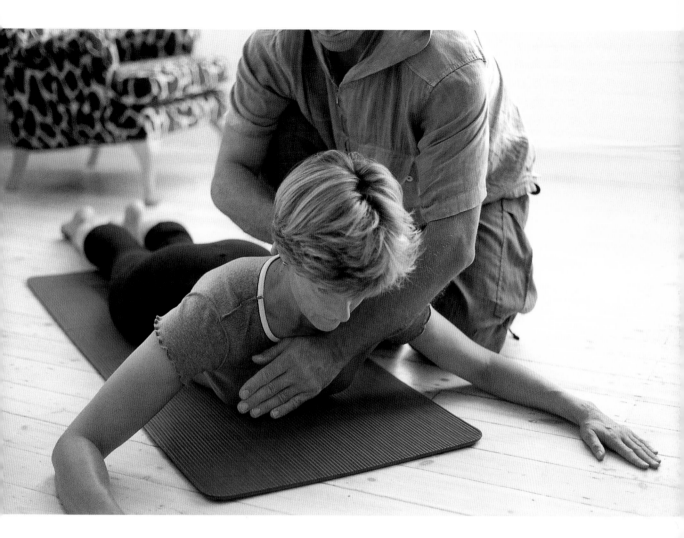

On the next **'out' breath**, lower your chest back down, one vertebra at a time, making sure that you don't squeeze your shoulder blades together.

Repeat 6–10 times.

watchpoints

– Make sure your elbows stay on the floor.
– Do not lift your lower ribs off the floor or compress the lower spine or neck.
– Always lengthen your spine.

3

aim

- To strengthen the lower back muscles.

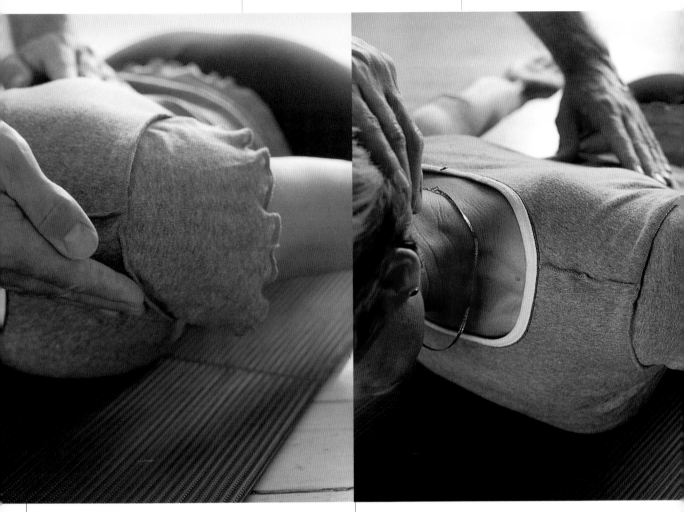

preparation

Begin in the same starting position as in The Cobra (see page 62), but place your arms flat at your sides with the palms of your hands facing up.

Make sure that your shoulders are square, not touching the mat.

Breathe in, pull up your pelvic floor, pull in your stomach muscles and squeeze the buttocks.

Breathing out, keeping your neck straight, lift your shoulders and pull with the lats towards your hips. Then lift your breastbone and hands off the floor.

Check that your hands are at the same level as the top of the buttocks, and your head is lifted about 10cm (4in) off the floor. You should be resting on your ribs, pubic bone and hip bones, and your abdominal muscles should be lifted.

1

back extension

2

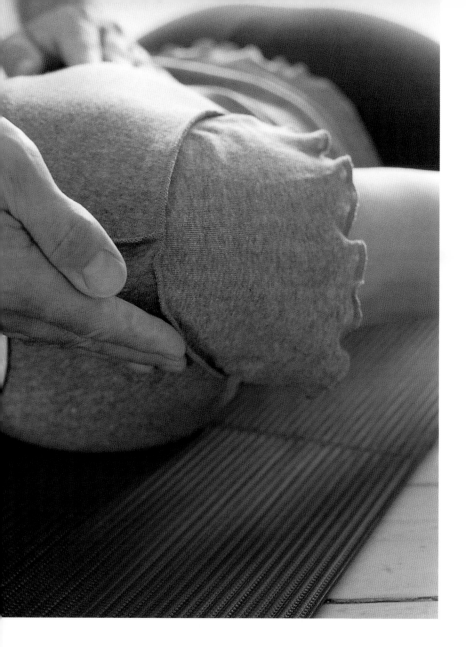

Breathe in as you come back down, bringing your shoulders back to their original position.

Repeat 6–10 times.

watchpoints

– Do not push the abdominal muscles out and do not lift too high.
– Do not arch the neck.
– Do not lift your legs.

3

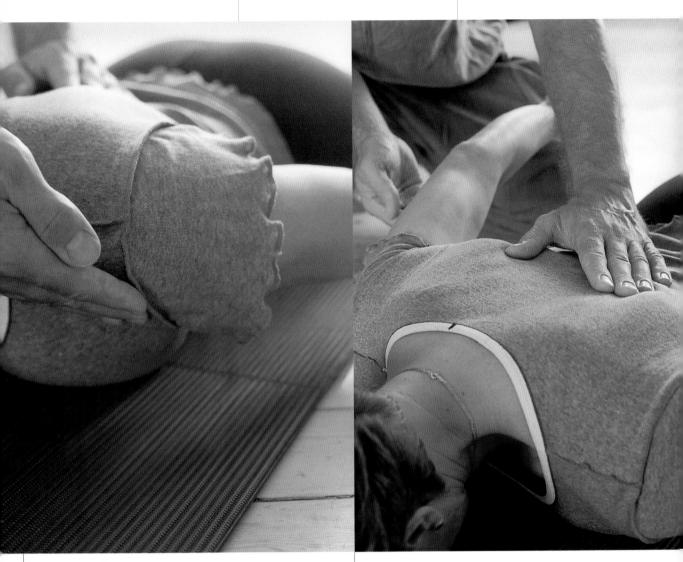

preparation

Begin in the same starting position as in the Back Extension (see page 64).

Breathe in, pull up your pelvic floor, pull in your stomach muscles and squeeze the buttocks.

Breathing out, pull with the lats towards your hips as before.

Lift your arms, using the triceps on the back of the arm, until they are slightly higher than the top of your shoulders.

Hold the position and **breathe in**.

1 arm lift

2

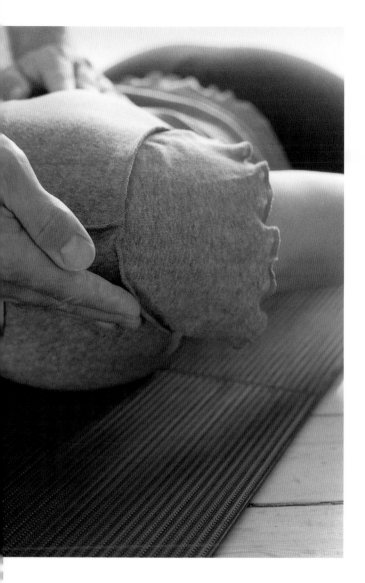

Breathing out, bring your arms and shoulders down to the mat, keeping your triceps working.

Repeat 6–10 times.

watchpoint

– Do not push your abdominals out.
– Do not squeeze your shoulder blades together.
– Keep your forehead on the floor.

3

aim

– To stretch the lower back.

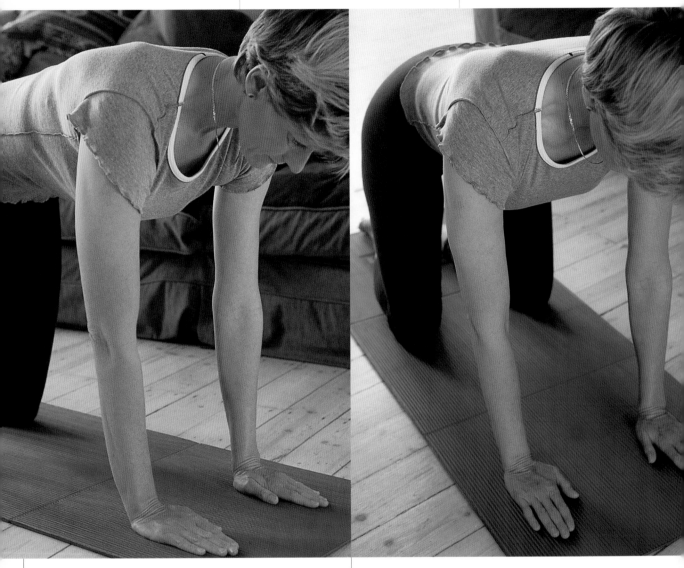

preparation

Begin on your hands and knees, making sure that your knees are hip-width apart.

Breathe in, pull up your pelvic floor and pull in your stomach muscles.

Breathing out, move your buttocks back as far as is comfortable for you.

Make sure you keep your arms straight, and that you are moving your buttocks back in a straight line.

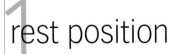

1 rest position 2

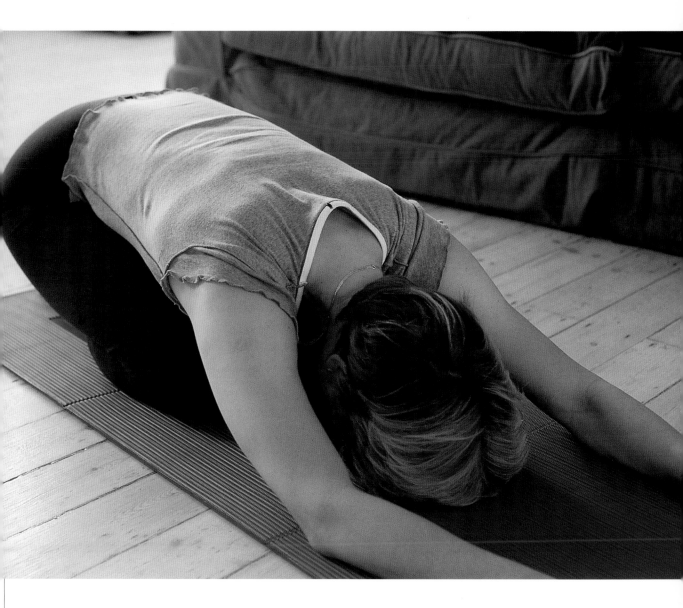

Rest in this position for **5 breaths**.

3

watchpoint
– If you have any problems with your knees, do not do this exercise.

aim
– To increase spinal articulation.

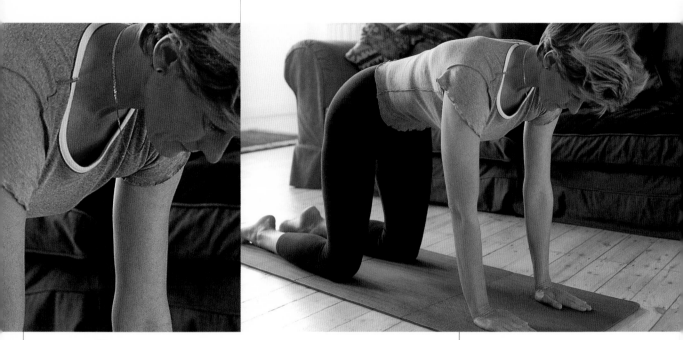

preparation

Start on your hands and knees again, making sure that your hands are beneath your shoulders and that your hips are above your knees.

Make sure that your back is flat, not tilted up or down.

Check that your head and neck are in alignment with your back, parallel to the floor.

Breathe in, sensing the breath coming in between your shoulder blades.

Pull up your pelvic floor and pull in your stomach muscles.

Breathing out, curl your tailbone underneath you, push into the heel of your hands and lift your breastbone, tucking your chin and then your head underneath.

Your back should now be rounded. Hold this position and **breathe in**.

1 the cat

2

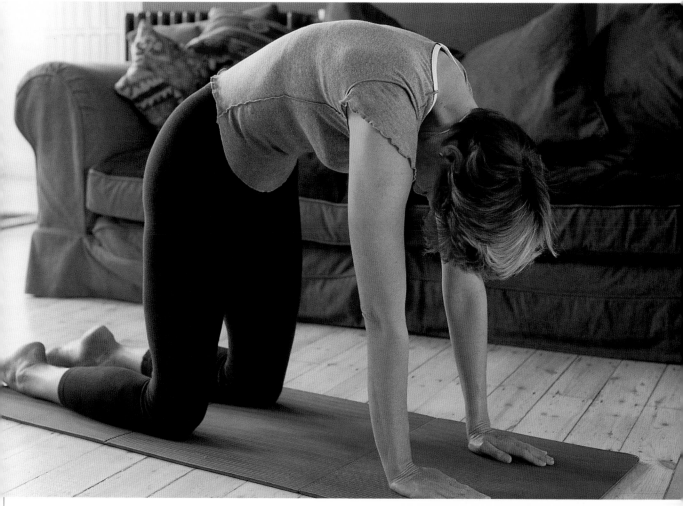

Breathe out and lower yourself back into the starting position by reversing the sequence, bringing your head back up to its position parallel with the floor followed by your chin and then your tailbone.

Repeat 3–6 times.

3

watchpoints
– Do not let your abdominal muscles go.
– Concentrate on lengthening the curve.

aim

– To stretch the Erector spinae.

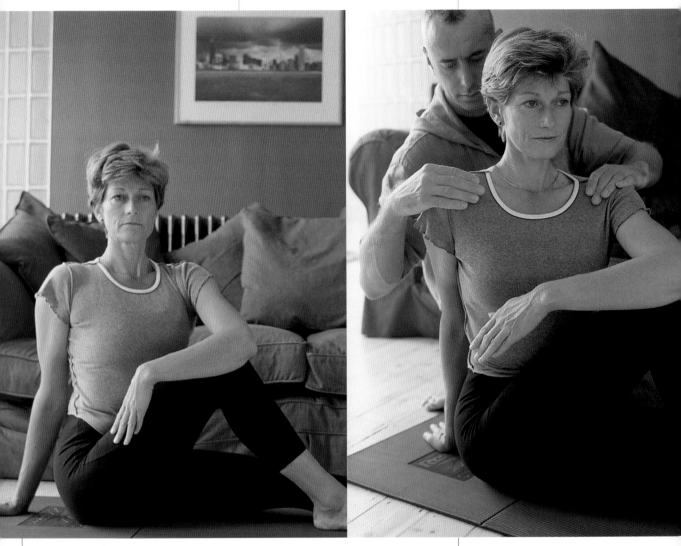

preparation

Begin by sitting on the mat with your legs in front of you. Raise your right knee, and put your right hand behind your back. Rest your left elbow on your right knee.

Breathe in, pulling up your pelvic floor, pulling in your stomach muscles and squeezing the buttocks, while lengthening the spine by pulling the vertebrae away from each other.

Breathing out, rotate your waist towards your raised leg.

Take a breath in and lengthen the spine.

Breathe out and rotate a little further.

1 sitting twist

2

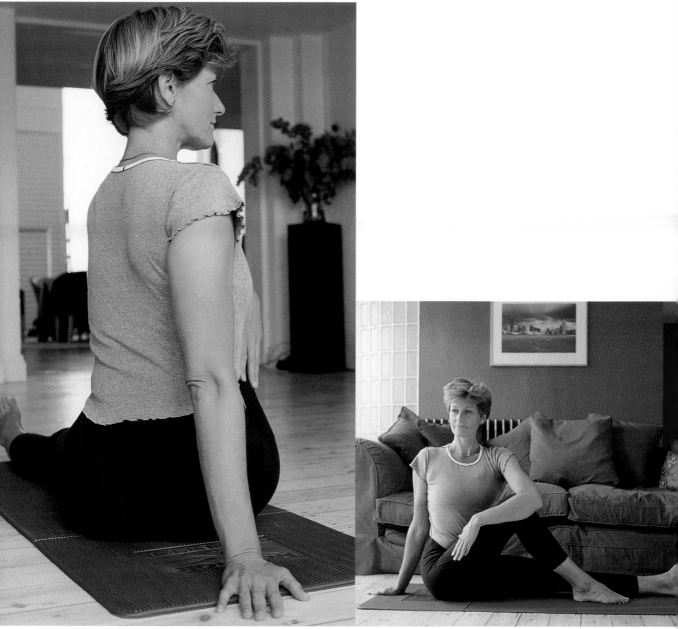

Breathe in as you rotate back
to the starting position.

Repeat 3 times each side.

3

watchpoints

– Keep your chin in line with the sternum.
– Keep your supporting arm straight.
– Do not collapse into your lower back.

aim

– To strengthen the Transversus
  abdominis and Rectus abdominis
  muscles.

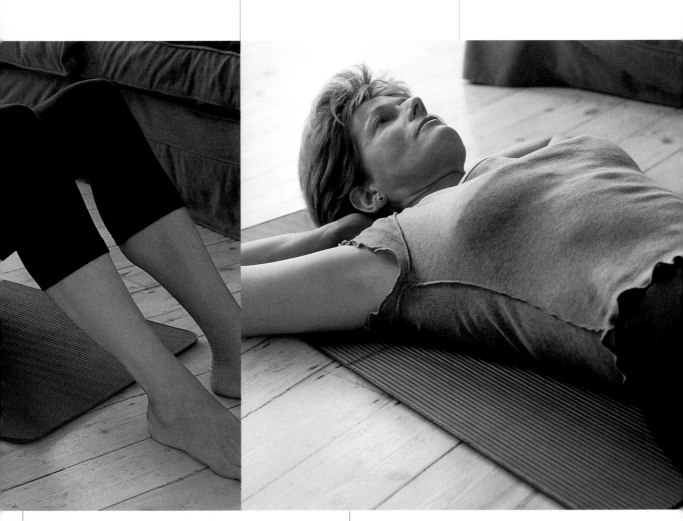

preparation

Begin by lying on the floor with your knees bent.
Your feet and knees should be hip-width apart.

Place your hands behind your head with your
elbows out to the side.

Breathe in, pull up your pelvic floor, pull in your
stomach muscles and squeeze your buttocks.

As you **breathe out,** imagine a cord pulling you
up from the centre of your chest.

1 abdominal lift   2

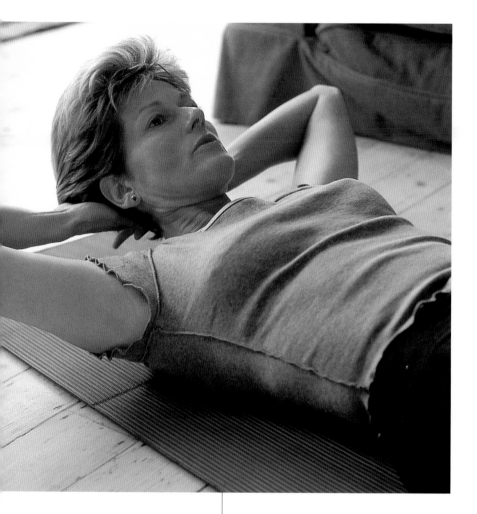

Raise your head off the mat. Your shoulders will rise a little, but the bottom of your shoulder blades should still touch the mat.

Breathe in as you come down, keeping your stomach muscles working.

Repeat 6–10 times.

3

4

watchpoints

– Do not move your pelvis or flatten your spine.
– When raising your head, your neck must not bend forwards.
– Support the weight of your head with your hands.

aim

- To strengthen the internal and external oblique muscles.

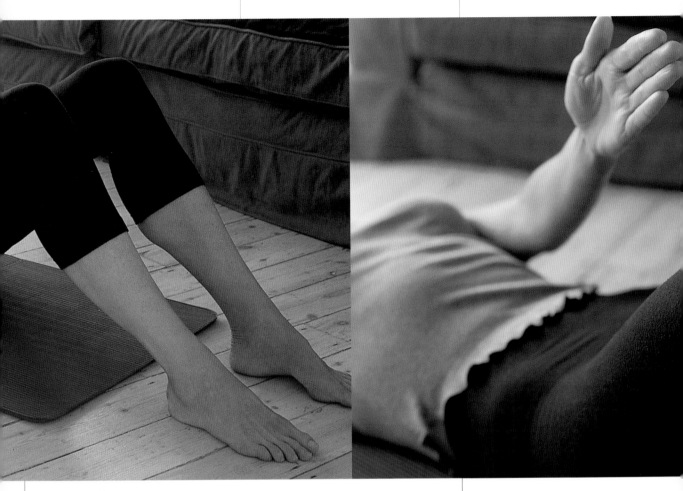

preparation

Begin by lying on your back with your knees bent and the cushion between your legs, but with only one hand behind your head.

Cross your other arm over your body, stretching it towards the opposite thigh.

Breathe in, pull up your pelvic floor and pull in your stomach muscles.

Breathing out, imagine a cord pulling your breastbone forward and at the same time rotate your body to the side.

If you start with your right hand behind your head and your left hand by your right leg, rotate towards the right side.

1 abdominal twist

2

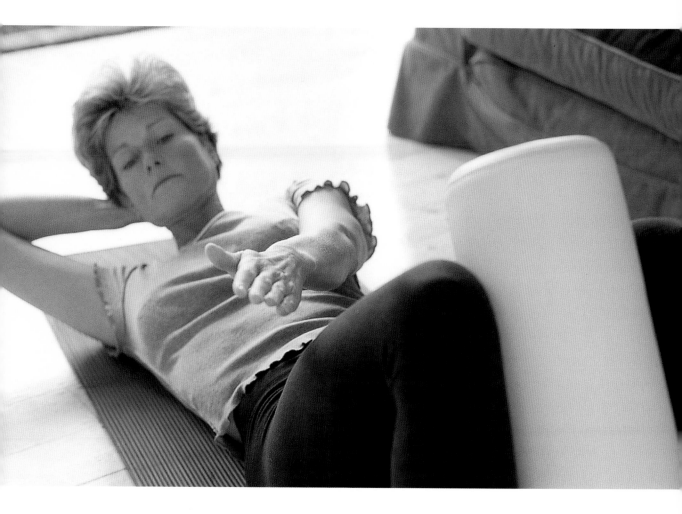

Breathe in and return to the starting position, keeping your stomach muscles working.

Repeat 3–6 times each side.

watchpoints

– Do not bend your neck.
– Do not let your legs move apart, remember to slightly squeeze the cushion.
– Do not let your hips lift off the floor.
– Keep your neck relaxed.

3

aim

– To strengthen the Transversus abdominis and Rectus abdominis muscles.

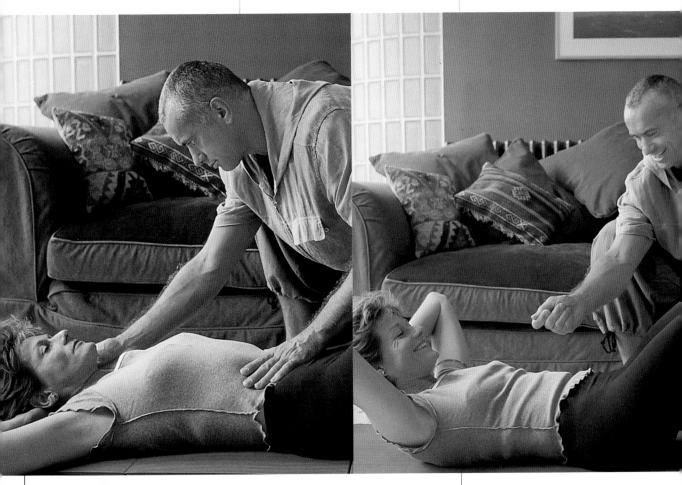

preparation

Begin in the same position as in the Abdominal Lift (see pages 74–75), but keep the knees and the feet together and have both hands behind the head. You do not need the cushion for this exercise.

Breathe in, pull up your pelvic floor and pull in your stomach muscles.

Breathe out and lift your breastbone as before.

1

2

abdominal curl with legs

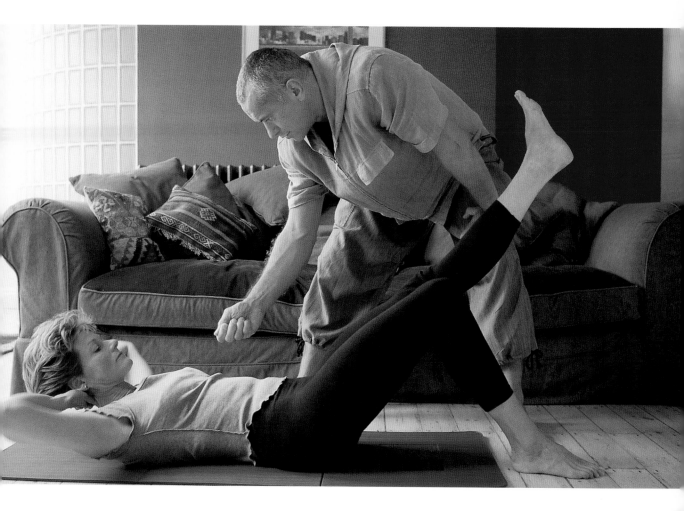

At the same time, lift one leg up from the knee.

Breathe in and return your head and leg to the starting position. Repeat this movement using your other leg.

Repeat 3–6 times each side.

3

watchpoints

– Do not allow your pelvis to move.
– Do not flatten your lower back.
– Do not bend your neck.
– Keep your neck relaxed.

For many people, the upper part of the body, including the chest, the back, the neck and the shoulders, is the area where the effects of poor posture are most keenly felt and also most visible.

In general, people tend to be closed up in the front of the upper body and have tightened chest muscles. This affects the posture and makes the shoulders round, causing problems in the upper back. In many cases, our sitting posture intensifies this problem. All too often, we slouch in a chair or sit hunched over a desk, allowing our shoulders to sag forward and our spine to become rounded. In these positions the head is badly supported and puts strain on the neck muscles. This in turn causes headaches and stiffness.

The following exercises reverse this process by opening the chest and lengthening the shoulder muscles. This provides a strong and upright support for the head.

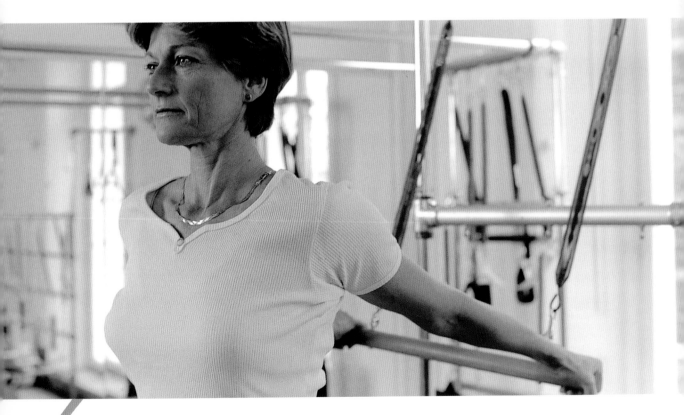

6 the upper body

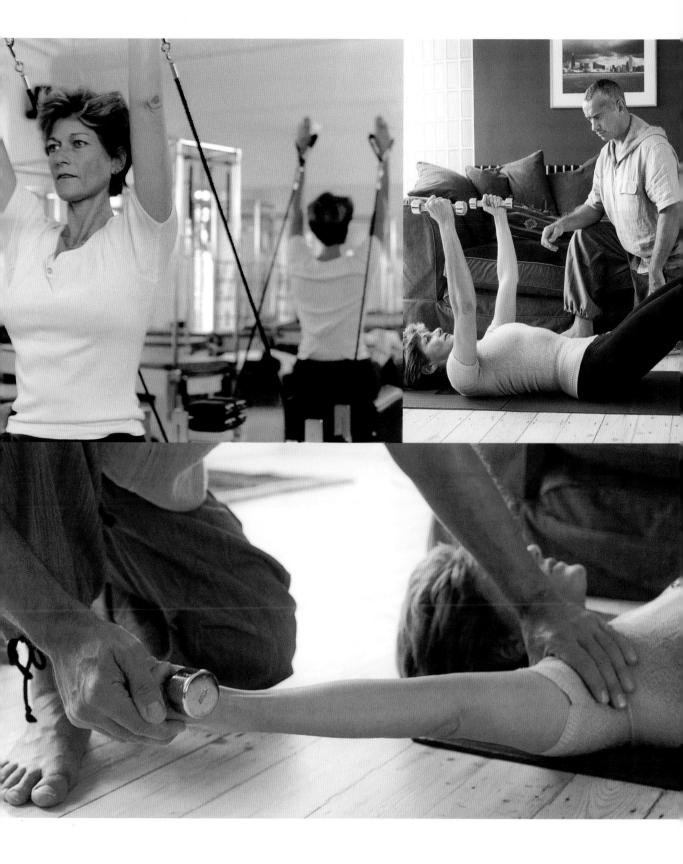

Working the Upper Body

Without the creation of a strong centre as emphasized in the Pilates Core Stabilization exercises, the upper body tends to collapse downwards, pulled by gravity and unsupported by a strong foundation. To combat this, we strengthen and lengthen the muscles in this area in order to keep ourselves upright. It is not surprising that the upper body is the place where we hold much of our tension. **What we need here is to release the tension, open up and stretch the upper body, and tone and strengthen the muscles so they will support us with ease.**

It is important to open up the chest because we need to breathe properly. The chest cavity houses the lungs and the heart, and without adequate room neither can function at optimum capacity. People with breathing problems such as bronchitis and asthma will often be those who are most closed up across the chest, as conditions like these tend to create a posture that attempts to compensate for the breathing difficulties. The effort involved in trying to breathe with blocked airways creates enormous tension in the upper back and tightness in the chest, which in turn makes the muscles shorter and tighter. But even people without breathing problems can be inclined to tight chest muscles because of poor posture.

The Pilates exercises in this section are specifically aimed at the chest and shoulder girdle, opening up the front of the chest, and consequently taking the strain away from the upper back and the shoulders. They involve the use of weights. You can do the exercises without weights, but their advantage is that they add extra resistance and lengthen the muscle more than if the exercise was done without them. It should be noted however, that people with osteoporosis should do the exercises without the use of weights.

The type of weights used in Pilates will not result in bulging muscles, as the weights are too light and the number of repetitions of each exercise is too low. Instead, they will help to give your muscles more definition, particularly in the upper arms, an area prone to loss of tone with age, regardless of body weight.

The shoulder joints are particularly prone to injury, as they articulate through a large range of movement. (It is for this reason that you should never lift a child up by the arm.) Partly because the joint is loose to allow free movement in a number of directions, there is an intricate arrangement of tendons and muscle keeping the shoulder joint in place. When we are young, the joint is kept well lubricated and the surrounding muscles and tendons are mobile because we use our arms and shoulders regularly. Unless we play sport or work in an occupation that demands regular use of the arms and shoulders we tend to limit their use as we get older. Also, injuries to the hands or forearm and conditions such as rheumatoid arthritis may mean that we move the arms less. All of these situations are likely to result in stiff joints and weak muscles. **One of the aims of Pilates exercises is to strengthen the muscles around the joints without putting any stress on the joints themselves.**

the upper body

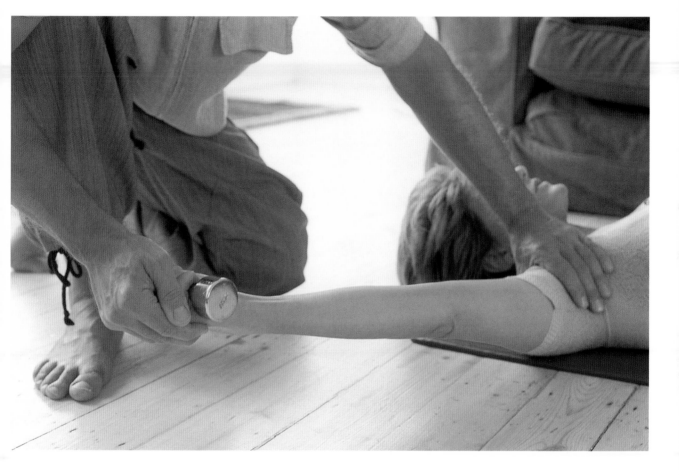

While the neck is an important part of the upper body, and also a very delicate one, it is not included in this section. The neck is particularly prone to holding tension and it also has to struggle to keep the head up. One of the reasons it is so prone to damage is that the weight of the head, some 5kg (11lb), is constantly compressing the cervical spine, which starts at the base of the skull. Because of this the neck muscles need to be regularly stretched and strengthened – exercises to do this are included in the Stretches chapter (see pages 124–5).

aim

– To open the chest and shoulders
and tone the chest muscles.

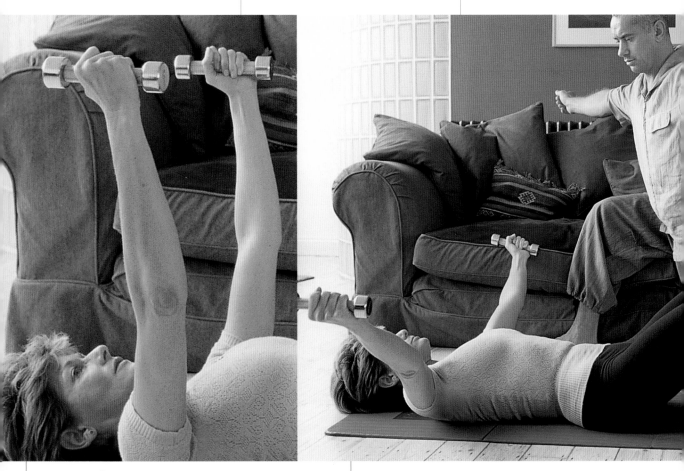

preparation

Begin by lying down with your knees bent,
holding a weight of 500g–1kg (1–2 lb) in each
hand, palms facing inward. Bring your arms up
above you, keeping them straight but without
locking your elbows.

Breathe in, pull up your pelvic floor and pull in
your stomach muscles.

Breathing out, lower your arms very slowly out
to your sides.

Hold the position and **take a small breath in**.

1

2

chest opener

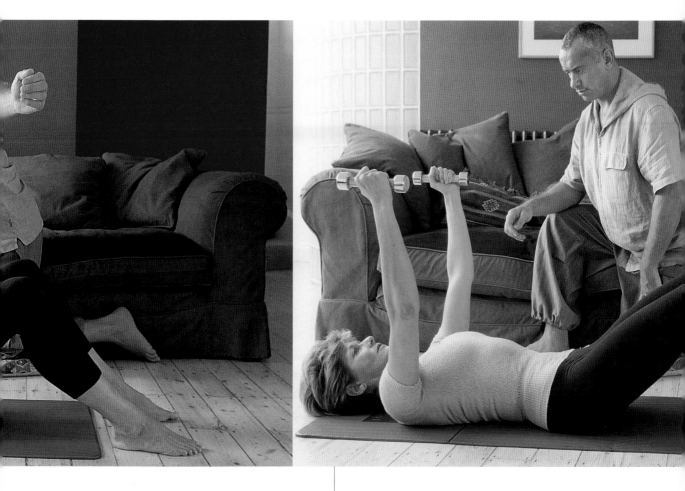

Breathing out again, bring your arms back up slowly, using your chest muscles to do the movement.

Repeat 6–10 times.

watchpoints
– Do not let go of your pelvic floor.
– Do not allow your lower back to arch.

3

aim

- To stretch the shoulders and strengthen the lats.

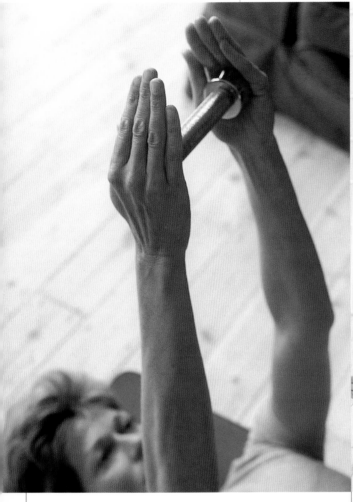

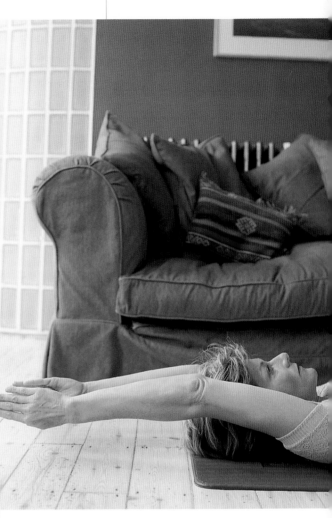

preparation

Begin by lying down with your knees bent and your arms raised, holding a weight held between your hands.

Breathe in, pull up your pelvic floor and pull in your stomach muscles.

Breathing out, slowly bring both your arms back over your head.

Hold the position and **breathe in**.

1rms over head 2

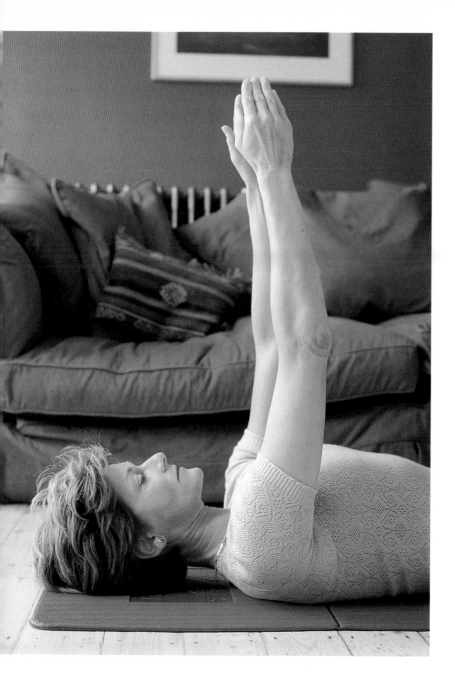

Breathing out, pull the muscles that run down
the side and back of the trunk towards your waist
as you bring your arms back up.

Repeat 6–10 times.

3

watchpoint

– Make sure your shoulders, your ribcage and your
back do not lift off the mat as you bring your arms
over your head. They must remain stable.

aim
– To mobilize the shoulders.

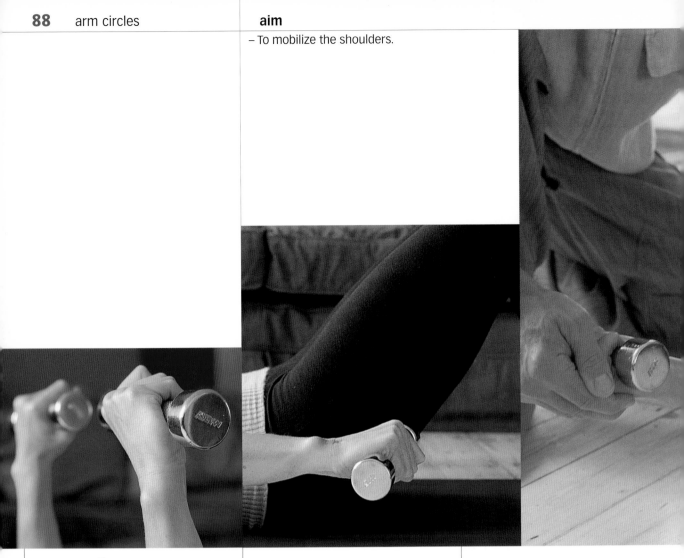

preparation

Begin in the same starting position as for Chest Opener (see pages 84–85), with knees bent and arms raised, a weight in each hand, but this time rotate your hands so that the palms are facing downwards.

Pull up your pelvic floor and pull in your stomach muscles.

Breathe in and bring your arms down beside your hips.

Rotate your hands so your palms face upwards.

Breathing out, circle both arms out to the sides horizontally, and up above the head, in line with your shoulders.

1 arm circles

2

3

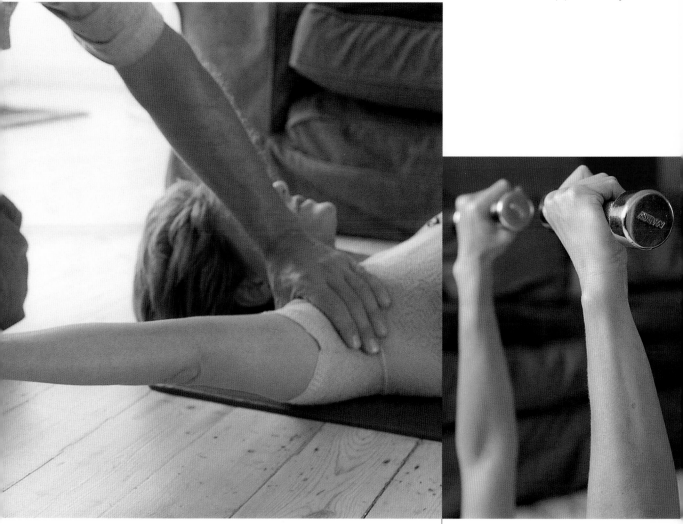

Breathing in, bring your arms up and over, lowering them back beside your hips.

Repeat 6–10 times, then reverse the direction.

watchpoint
– Do not lock your elbows. Always keep them slightly rounded and soft.

4

aim

– To strengthen and lengthen the
  Rhomboid muscles.

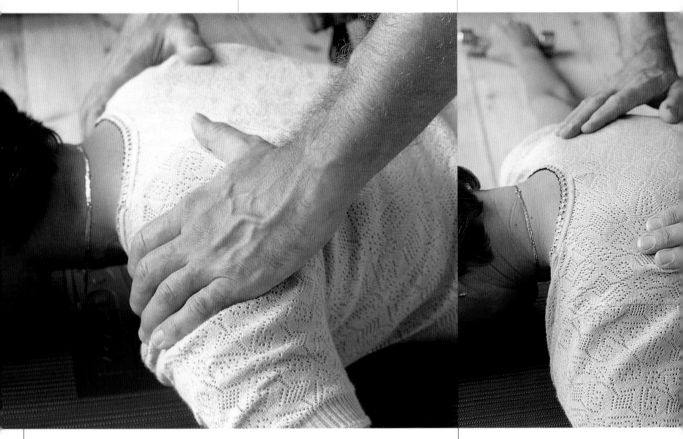

preparation

Begin by lying face down on the mat, your arms out to the side and
your hands (holding the weights) slightly below shoulder level.

Breathe in, pull up your pelvic floor and pull in your stomach
muscles.

Breathe out and lengthen
your arms to the side.

1 upper back strengthener   2

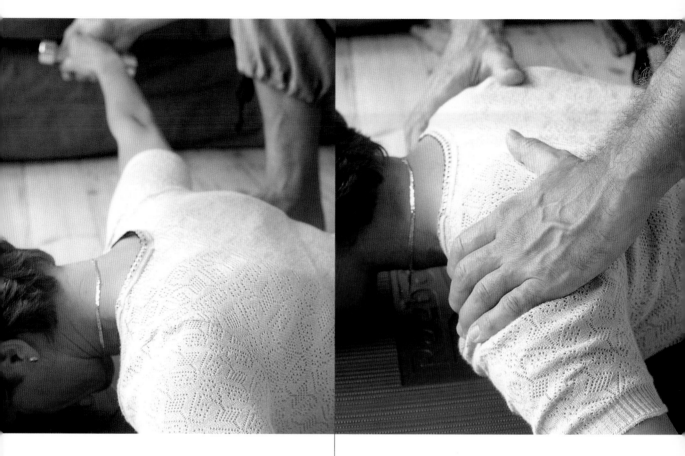

Lift your hands and arms about 10cm (4in) off
the floor.

Breathe in and slowly lower your arms to
the floor.

Repeat 6–10 times.

watchpoints
– Do not squeeze your shoulder blades together.
– As in all the upper body exercises, keep your
  neck and shoulders relaxed.

3

4

Legs, and particularly feet, are our support and also our connection with the earth. In Eastern philosophies, earth energy, which is essential for vitality, enters through points on the soles of the feet. Lack of mobility in the feet can block the flow of that energy and so affect our health. On a more physical level, stiffness in the feet and ankles impedes movement, such as walking, and ultimately affects the alignment of the entire body. For example, an ankle problem can lead to back ache if, when compensating for physical discomfort, we force our bodies into unhealthy positions. In this way, discomfort moves up through the legs and into the spine.

Our legs are a source of physical freedom and independence. They give us certain choices: to run away from danger or to walk towards friends. When our lower limbs are not working properly, our mobility, and often our choices, become limited. But with regular exercise, our legs will support us.

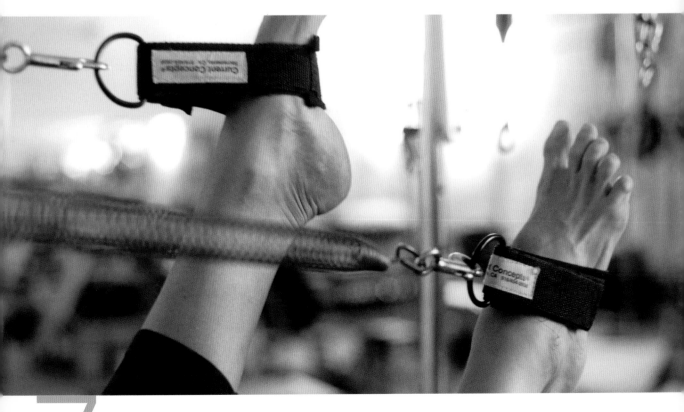

7
legs

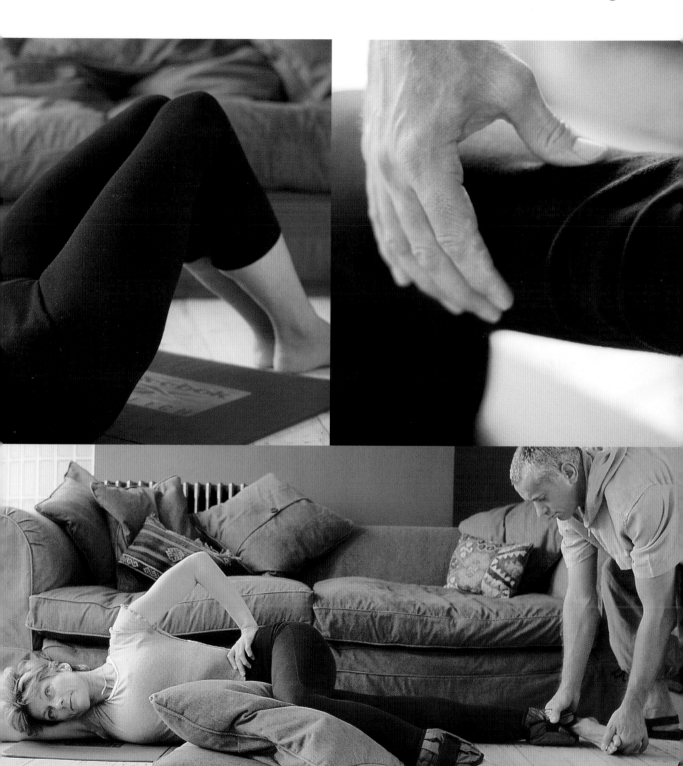

Legs and Feet – Our Support

The most important reasons for exercising the lower limbs are:

- **to strengthen and lengthen the muscles**
- **to preserve or increase joint mobility**
- **to increase circulation**

Circulation is included here because the upward flow of blood in the legs towards the heart is one of the most difficult feats for the body to accomplish, as blood moves against the force of gravity. It is the smooth action of muscles and joints in the leg that helps the blood flow upwards, but if the legs are underused it is apt to pool in the veins, creating little pockets and stretching the vein itself. The result is varicose veins, which in some cases causes discomfort. Certain people are genetically predisposed to the condition, while others, such as hairdressers and dentists, may suffer due to the conditions in which they work. Varicose veins are also associated with pregnancy. There are simple ways of counteracting the effects of constant standing. Wearing shoes that allow you to flex your toes regularly will assist circulation, as it is the feet muscles and those in the lower back of the leg that primarily push the blood upwards. This will also help aching legs in general.

Another preventive measure is to sit during break times with your feet raised to hip height, or even higher if possible, as this will help blood flow.

Included in the exercises for the lower body are ones that focus on the gluteal muscles, or buttocks. Massage therapists will tell you that many people hold a lot of tension in this muscle and that is why, during a massage, they work very hard to release that tension. The gluteal muscles play an important part in supporting the upper body and in helping us to stand up straight. Also, as we sit so much, the gluteal muscles do not get used as often as they should. Exercising these muscles will lift and firm them, improving the shape of the buttocks and the posture at the same time.

We tend to use our quadriceps most, and it is these muscles in the front of the thigh on which conventional exercise focuses when working the legs. However, the quadriceps are not postural muscles and do not support the pelvis. Instead, it is the inner thigh and hamstring muscles attached to the knee joint and going up under the pelvis that provide a supporting platform for the pelvis. When lengthened and strengthened, these leg muscles provide postural stability. Many people have shortened hamstring muscles. This is also true of the inner thigh muscles. However, when trying to lengthen these muscles, many people work them through only one dimension. As a result, there is no change through the entire muscle group and so the effort is wasted. Pilates exercises emphasize working through the three dimensions, so that progress is made in lengthening the muscle group and ensuring that it does not return to its original, shortened state.

Exercising the legs will also help to prevent, and to get rid of, cellulite, which mostly affects women. This

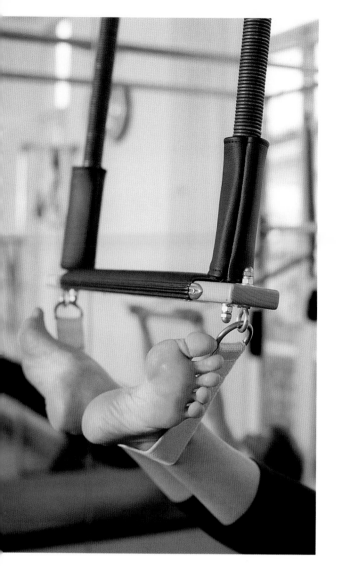

the form of lymphatic drainage and aromatherapy is recommended for treating the problem, but diet and exercise are two methods of self-help.

Leg Exercises

The aim of these leg exercises is to work the medial gluteal, or buttock, muscles and the thighs. If possible, buy a pair of leg weights from a sports shop. They should weigh about 1kg (2lb 4oz) each and strap around your ankles. Most leg weights are adjustable, so that you can decrease or increase their weight according to your ability. However, all the exercises here can be done without using leg weights. Remember that it is better to work with lighter weights and good technique than to keep strapping on extra kilos.

condition does not discriminate – it appears regardless of body weight, so being thin will not protect you from it. Men's muscles account for about 42 per cent of their body weight, and fat for only 18 per cent. In women, muscle accounts for only 36 per cent of body weight, and fat for 28 per cent, hence the problem. A higher fat to muscle ratio provides more opportunity for cellulite to appear.

There are no easy cures for cellulite, which consists of a build-up of toxins in the fatty tissues. Most experts are agreed that only changes in diet combined with exercise will remove the 'orange peel' effect, which is usually most visible in the upper thigh area. Massage in

aim

– To strengthen the middle buttock muscles and the outer thigh.

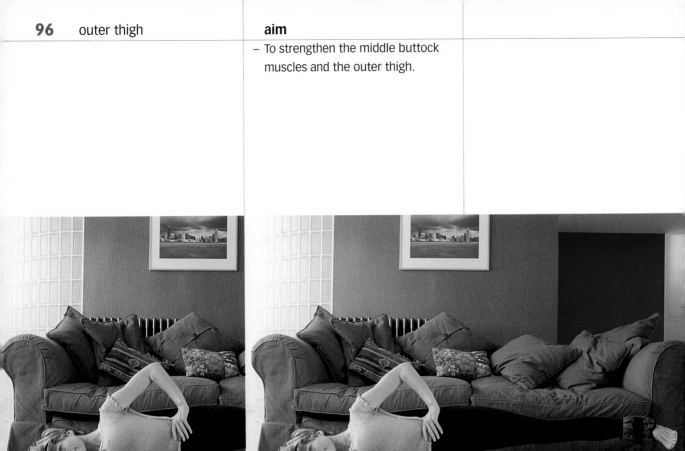

preparation

Begin by lying down on your right side. Bend your left arm and rest your hand on your hip bone. Bend your right leg in front of you.

Raise your right arm above your head, palm facing up, and rest your head on your arm.

Flex both your feet so they are at right angles to your legs, and lengthen your left leg without moving your hips.

Breathe in, pull up your pelvic floor and pull in with your stomach muscles.

Breathing out, lift your left leg, feeling your buttock muscles squeezing together.

1 outer thigh

2

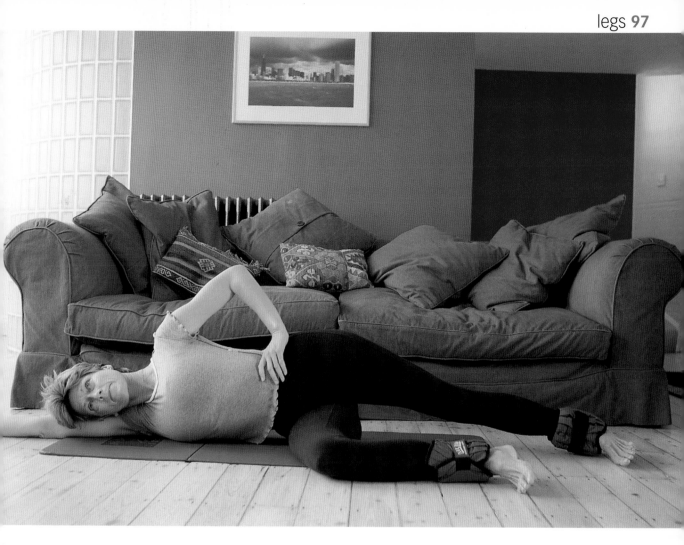

Breathe in and lower your leg to the starting position.

Repeat 6–10 times each side.

watchpoints

– Work your pelvic floor, stomach and buttock
muscles on both the in and out breaths.
– Do not arch your lower back or allow your waist
to shorten.
– Do not allow your lower ribs to push forward.

3

aim

– To strengthen the inner thigh.

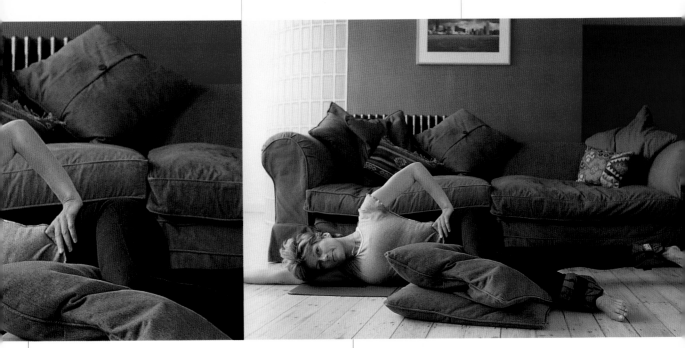

preparation

Begin by lying on one side again, but now bend your top leg and bring it in front of you. Put two pillows under this leg to support it and prevent you rolling your upper body forward.

Place your hand on your uppermost hip and flex your feet as for the Outer Thigh exercise (see pages 96–97).

Breathe in, pull up your pelvic floor, pull in your stomach muscles and squeeze your buttocks together.

Breathing out, lengthen your lower leg without moving your hip and raise it 15cm (6in) off the floor.

1 inner thigh

2

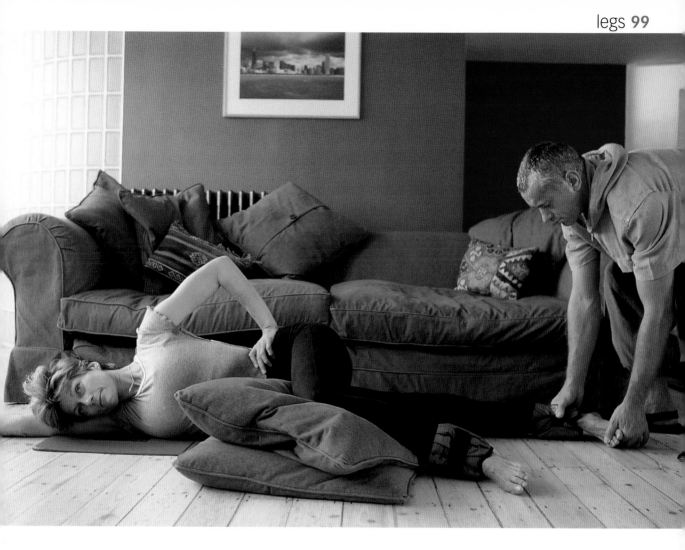

Breathe in and lower your leg.

Repeat 6–10 times each side.

watchpoints

– Work your pelvic floor, stomach and buttock
muscles on both the 'in' and 'out' breaths.
– Do not arch your lower back.
– Do not rotate your leg.
– Relax your neck.

3

aim

– To strengthen the hamstrings and
Gluteus maximus.

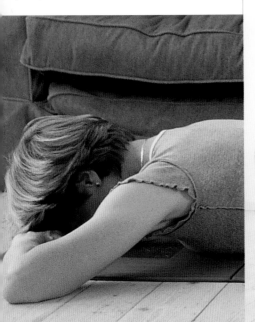
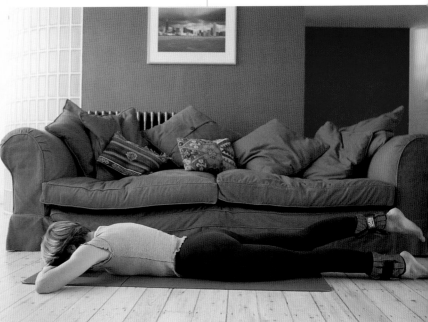

preparation

Begin by lying on your stomach
with your forehead resting on
your hands and your elbows
wide. If you have a sensitive
lower back, put a cushion
under your stomach.

Breathe in, pulling up your
pelvic floor and pulling in with
your stomach muscles.

Breathing out, raise one leg 10cm (4in) off the
floor, keeping it straight as you do so. Feel your
hamstring and buttock muscles working.

1 hamstring lift 2

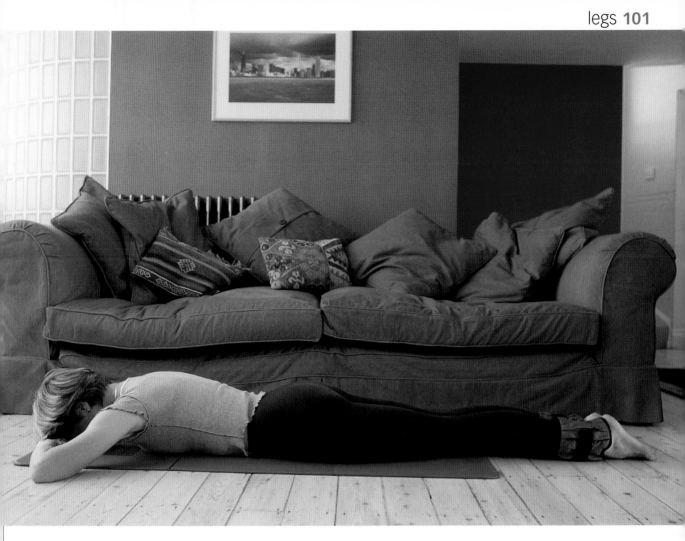

Breathing in, slowly lower your leg to the floor.

Repeat 6–10 times with each leg.

3

watchpoints
– Do not arch your lower back or push out your stomach.
– Keep your neck and shoulders relaxed.

aim

– To build longer, leaner hamstring muscles.

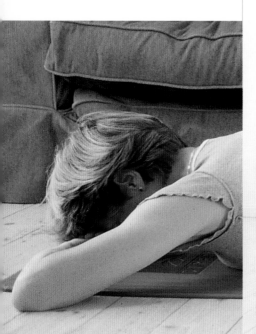

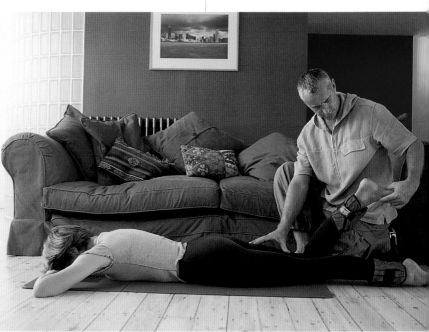

preparation

Begin in the same starting position as for the Hamstring Lift (see page 100).

Pull up your pelvic floor, pull in your stomach muscles and squeeze the buttocks.

Breathing in, bend one leg at the knee and bring the heel up towards your buttocks.

1 hamstring curl 2

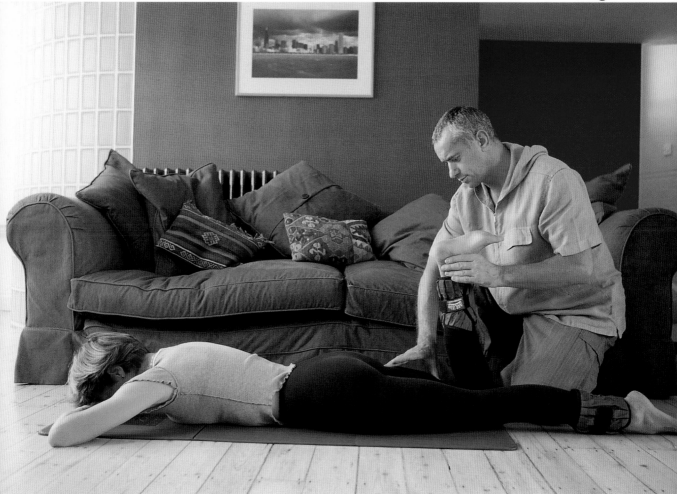

Breathing out, slowly lower your leg to the floor,
lengthening the hamstring.

Repeat 6–10 times with each leg.

watchpoints

– As you breathe out and lower your legs, focus your
  awareness on lengthening your hamstring muscles.
– Do not arch your lower back.
– Relax your neck and shoulders.

3

aim

– To tone and lift the Gluteus
maximus.

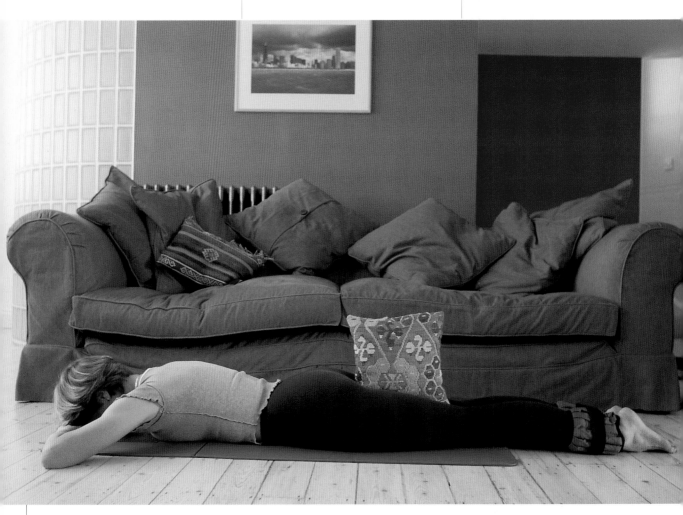

preparation

Lie down on your stomach. Place the pillow or
cushion between your thighs. Rest your forehead
on your hands, elbows wide.

Breathe in, pull up your pelvic floor and pull in
your stomach muscles.

1 buttock squeeze

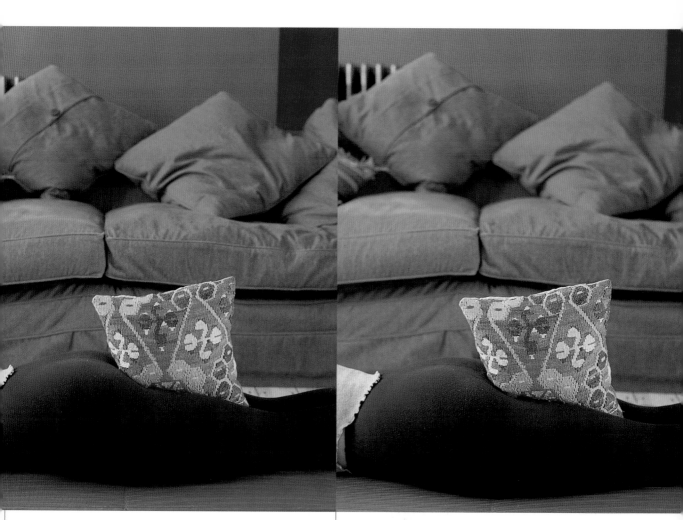

Breathing out, squeeze your thighs and buttocks together, and hold for a count of 6.

Breathe in and release your thigh and buttock muscles.

Repeat 6–10 times.

variation

Begin in the same starting position but rotate your legs outward so that your heels turn towards each other, then continue as before.

2

3

How many mornings do you wake up and instinctively feel like a good stretch even before you put a foot out of bed? Quite often, your whole body moves into that stretch, elongating your back, your arms and your legs, but without you consciously willing them. You might even yawn while you do it – another reflex action. Stretching your body like this feels pleasurable, but how good is it for you?

Joseph Pilates formed his theory of fitness based on the premise that our physical movements most benefited our health when they were conscious actions serving our will. So whether we are walking, sitting, turning or stretching, we should always direct our movements, clear in our minds as to exactly what we are doing and how advantageous it will be to us. Only then will we see the benefit.

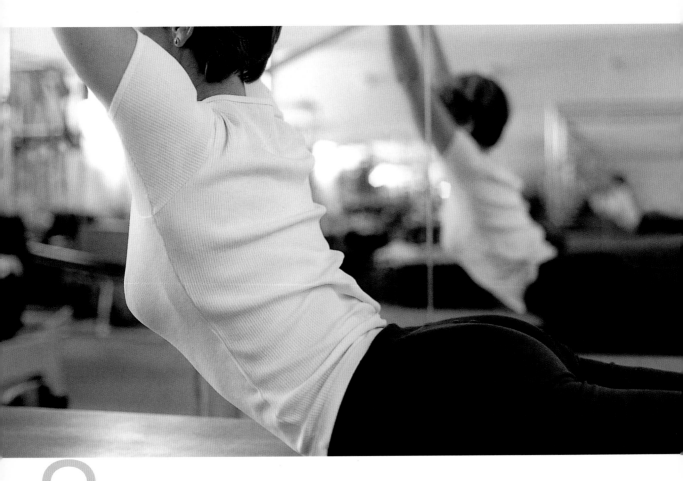

8 stretches

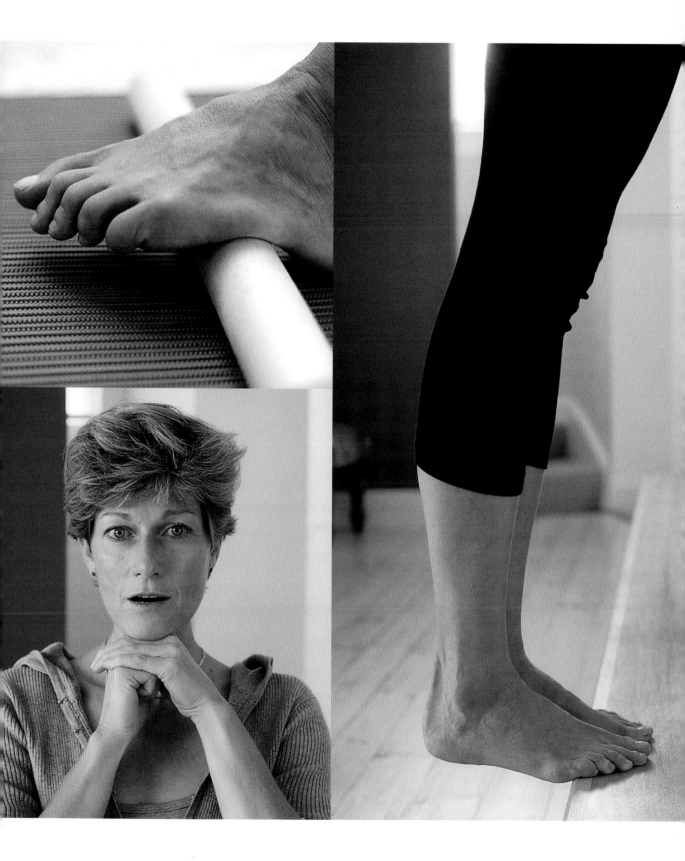

Stretching

Stretching helps to lengthen the muscles and to relax them. They stretch most effectively after they have been warmed up, which is why this sequence of stretches comes at the end of the exercise plan.

If we think of our muscles as having the same qualities as an elastic band, it is easier for us to understand the aim of doing stretches. Too much tension tightens our muscles and makes us feel tired and depressed. Relieving the muscle tension by stretching brings back elasticity, and aids muscle/joint harmonization. It also helps us to feel mentally more relaxed and therefore alert. **It is only in the last 50 years that the relationship between muscle tension and mental states has been recognized and properly researched.** The work of people like Joseph Pilates and Frederick M. Alexander (1869–1955), who developed the Alexander Technique, has contributed to a greater understanding of this.

When we are doing exercises we are contracting the muscles, as described earlier. Following this with stretches helps to make the muscles more elastic, and this in turn helps them to contract more easily. Think again of a rubber band. If you are given a cold and stiff rubber band, it is difficult to stretch it out. If you warm the rubber band a little and keep pulling it gently, it will gradually expand more and more. It will also snap back more easily once it has been warmed, softened and stretched. This is what you are doing with your muscles when you exercise and stretch.

Tight muscles cause a number of problems, and as the muscles are interconnected, an injury or condition may not arise in the area of tightness, but instead in an area connected to it. For example, lower back injuries can result from tight hamstring muscles, which are not uncommon. Tight hamstrings restrict mobility and result in the lower back also being tight. If the hamstrings are very tight, they pull on the pelvis, creating postural problems. Also, if the hip flexor is tight it too pulls on the pelvis. When these are combined, the pelvis is constantly being pulled out as if it was the centre knot in a tug-of-war. Similarly, if one leg is tighter than the other, the pelvis will be pulled by a different tension on each side. This creates uneven hips.

Although our feet and ankles bear our weight, the calf muscles are our first stage of muscular support. Most people have tight calf muscles and this can affect the back muscles.

Frequently, the jaw holds a lot of tension. This is a direct result of stress because we clench our teeth, literally and metaphorically, in response to constant irritation from our environment. Very often this clenching is an automatic reaction and we may not even realise what we are doing. Tension in the jaw can move into the neck and shoulders and from there into the back.

stretches

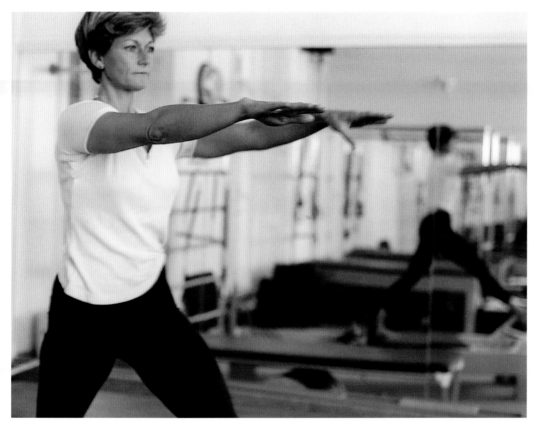

Pain

Stretching the muscles should feel comfortably uncomfortable. The sensation should be one of stretching, not one of tearing. If you experience a hot, shooting pain then you should stop the exercise immediately, otherwise you are likely to cause damage.

If you have not exercised for some time and are stiff and tight, you may experience some degree of pain when performing stretches. However, if you have worked through the Core Stabilization programme prior to stretching, you should find that the exercises that follow are much easier as the earlier exercises will have warmed up the muscles and already stretched them out somewhat. If you are in any doubt about the pain you are experiencing, consult a doctor and your Pilates teacher, if you have one.

aim

– To lengthen the hamstrings and stretch the lower back.

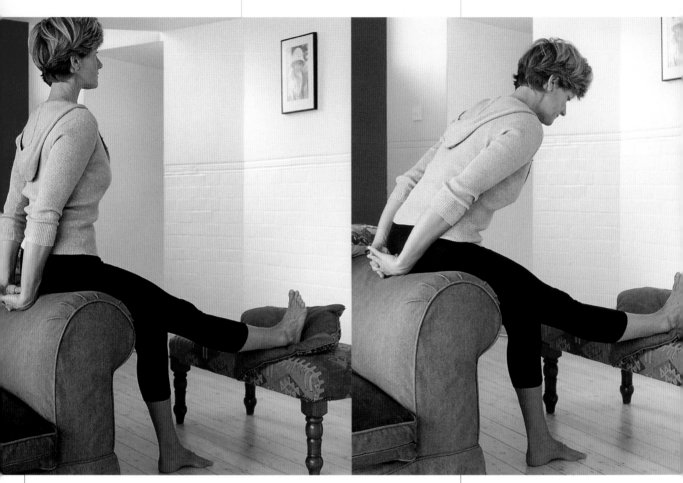

preparation

Place your buttocks on the edge of a desk, or the arm of a sofa, just enough to support your pelvis.

Place a low stool in front of you and put the heel of one foot on it. Make sure that the stool is close enough for you not to have to stretch your leg out to reach it.

Flex the supported foot upwards. Put your hands behind your back, but do not use them to support your weight.

Lengthen your spine and keep your chest open.

Breathe in, pull up your pelvic floor and pull in your stomach muscles.

Keeping your back straight, **breathe out** and bend over from the hips as far as you can while still keeping your back straight.

Hold the position for **5 long, slow breaths**.

1 hamstring stretches 2

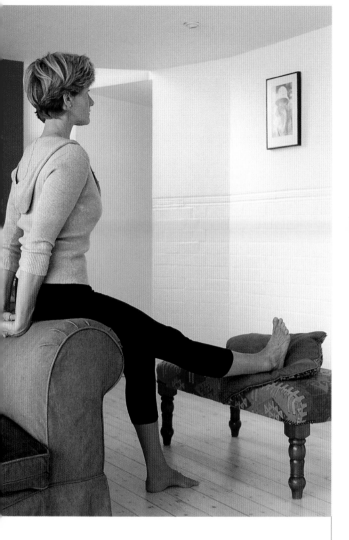

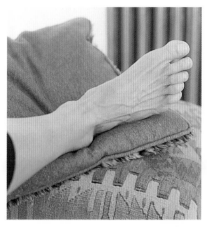

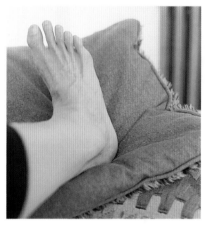

Breathe out and come back up.

Repeat 5 times for each leg.

watchpoints

– Do not bend your neck.

– Keep your shoulders open and relaxed.

– Do not twist your hips or rotate your spine.

With the working foot turned out, you can work on stretching your buttock and outer hamstring muscles.

By turning the foot in, you can stretch the inner part of your hamstring.

3

variation

aim

– To lengthen the calf muscles.

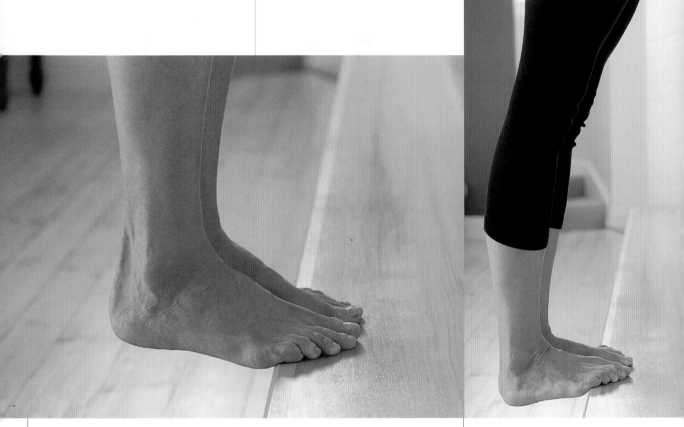

preparation

Standing and holding onto a support with one hand, place the balls of your feet on the step.

Pull up your pelvic floor and pull in your stomach muscles. Check that your back is not arched.

Breathing out, lower your heels as far as they will go.

Hold the position for **6 breaths**.

1 calf stretch

2

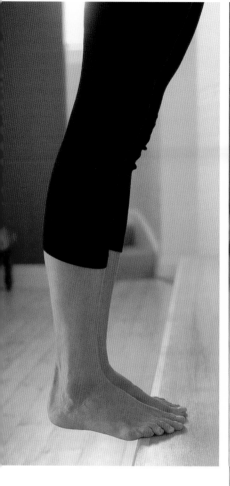

Lift your heels again so that
your feet are parallel with
the floor.

Repeat 3–6 times.

Repeat the exercise first with
your feet turned out, and then
with your feet turned in.

watchpoints

– Do not arch your back.
– If you feel strain in your lower back only do
  4 repetitions, and use your stomach and
  buttock muscles to support you.

3

variation

aim

– To create supple buttock muscles, which play an important role in the health of the lower back.

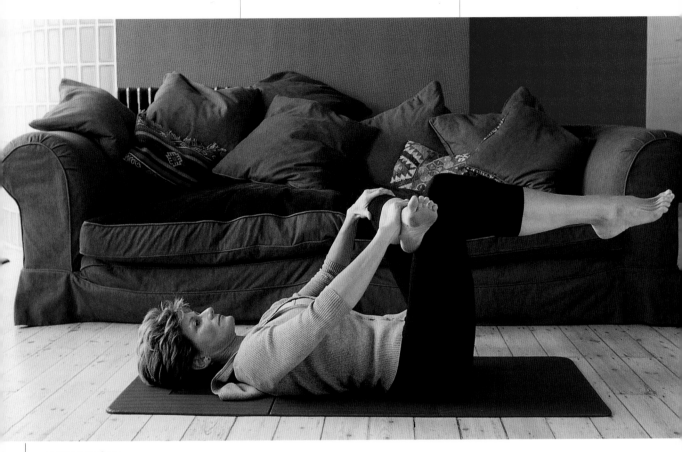

preparation

Lie down on the mat with your right hip and knee bent at right angles.

Cross your left leg over and support the ankle on the right knee or just above it.

Hold this ankle while keeping your head flat on the floor. If necessary you can put a towel or small pillow under your head.

Breathe in, pull up your pelvic floor and pull in your stomach muscles.

buttock stretches

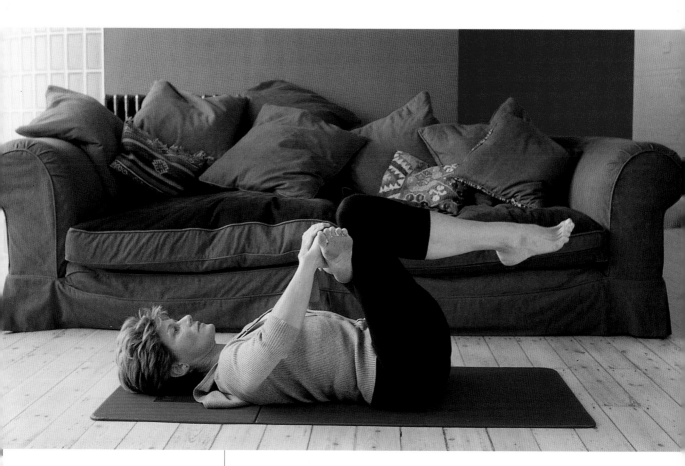

Breathing out, pull the left ankle up towards you slightly. You will feel the left buttock muscles stretch.

Hold this position for **5 long, slow breaths**.

Repeat with the other leg.

Repeat 3–6 times each side.

2

3

watchpoints
– Do not lift your tailbone.
– Do not twist your pelvis.

aim

– To lengthen the Quadriceps.

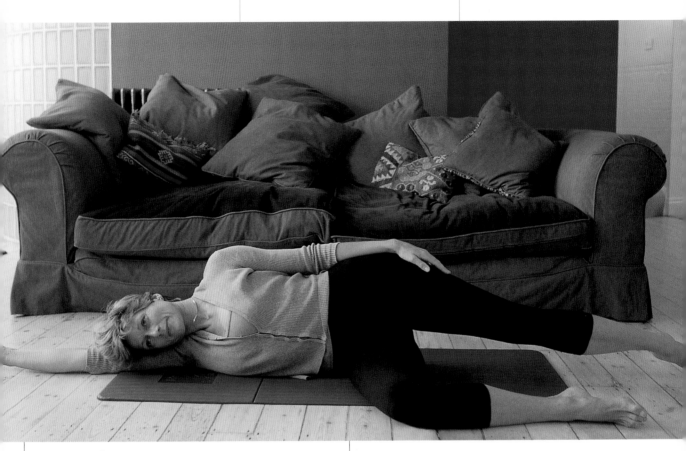

preparation

Lie down on one side and bend your lower leg up towards your trunk. The higher up you can place it, the better the muscles will stretch.

Breathe in, pull up your pelvic floor and pull in your stomach muscles.

Breathing out, reach down and take hold of the ankle of your upper leg and pull it up behind you, towards the buttocks. Feel the quadricep muscles in the front of your thighs stretching.

quadriceps stretches

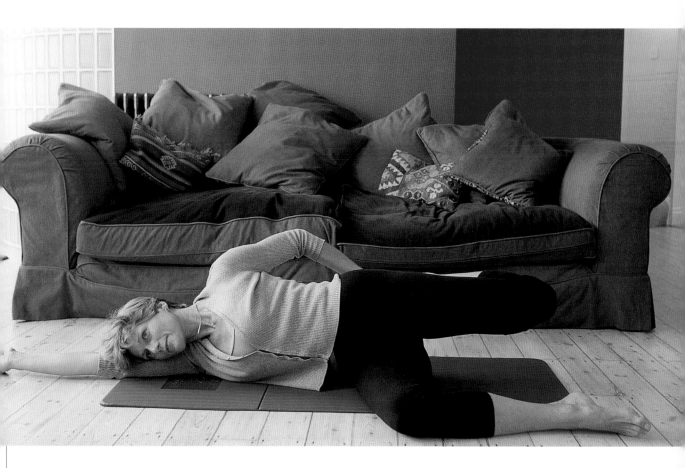

Hold the position for **5 breaths**, then release your ankle and bring your leg back down.

Repeat 3–6 times each side.

3

watchpoints

– Do not arch your back.
– Slightly tuck your pelvis forward. This will protect your back and increase the stretch in your quadriceps.

aim

– To create supple hip flexors.

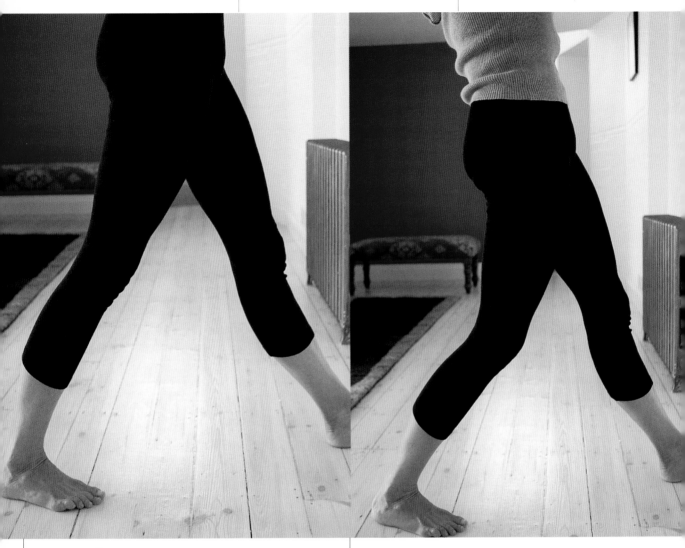

preparation

Stand up facing a wall. Bring your left leg close to the wall, while keeping both legs straight.

Put both hands on the wall, but do not keep your arms rigidly straight.

Breathe in, pull up your pelvic floor and pull in your stomach muscles.

Tuck your pelvis underneath, bend your right leg and feel the stretch in the front of the hip of your right leg.

1 hip stretches 2

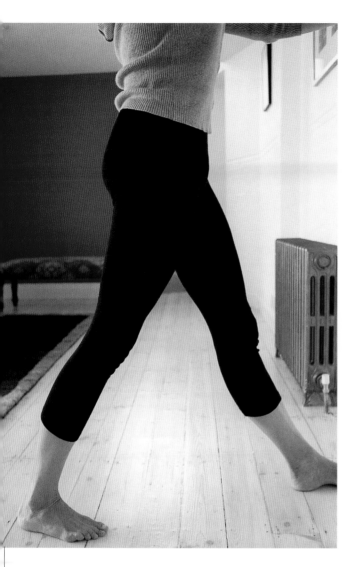

Hold the position for **5 breaths**.

Repeat 3–6 times each side.

3

aim

– To stretch across the front of the chest.

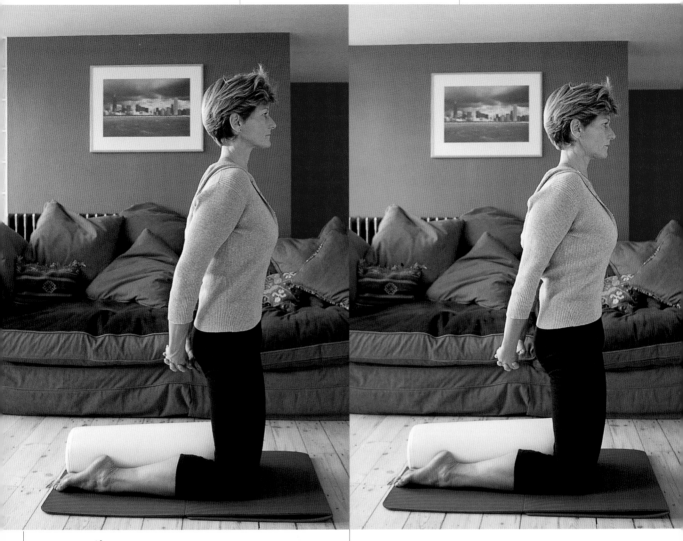

preparation

Kneel with a cushion between your knees and calves.

Squeeze the cushion and clasp your hands behind your back at the level of the buttocks.

Breathe in, pull up your pelvic floor and pull in your stomach muscles.

Breathe out, pull your shoulders back and squeeze your shoulder blades together, imagining that you are pulling them back from the centre of your breastbone.

1

2

shoulder stretch 1

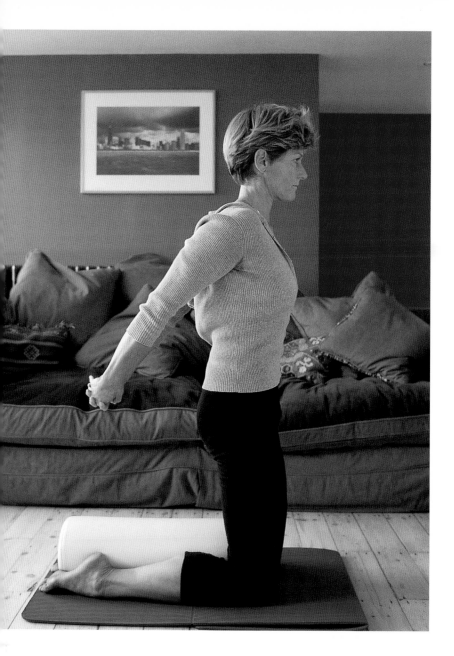

Stretch your clasped hands away from your buttocks.

Hold the position for **3 breaths**.

Repeat 3–6 times.

3

aim

– To lengthen the lats and stretch the middle of the back.

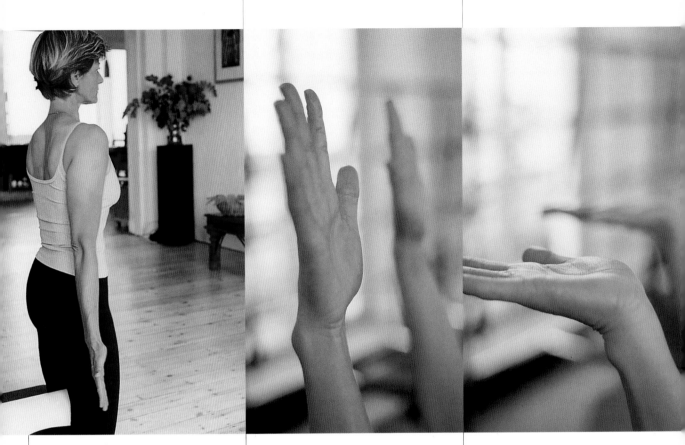

preparation

Kneel as in Shoulder Stretch 1 (see page 120), but with your hands by your sides, palms facing forward.

Pull up your pelvic floor and pull in your stomach muscles.

Breathing in, raise your hands above your head, your palms facing forward.

When lifting your arms, lift them from beneath the lats.

Lift your shoulders and shoulder blades, and flex your hands back.

1

shoulder stretch 2

3

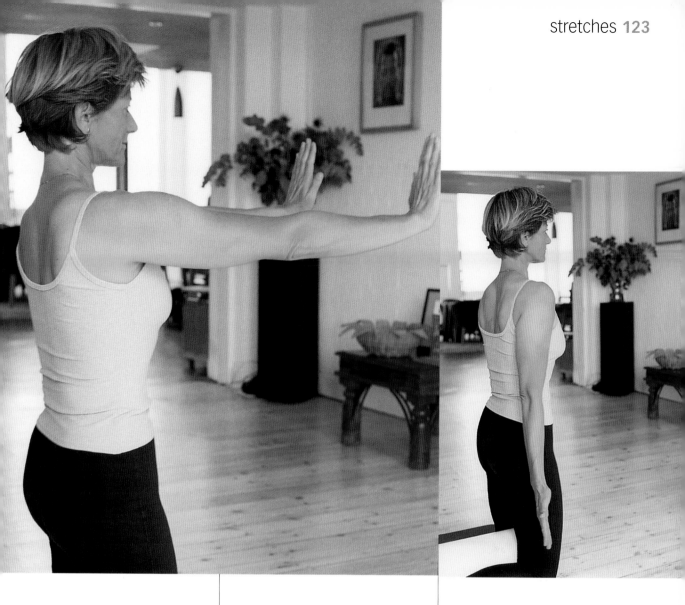

Breathing out, keeping your shoulders lifted and your hands flexed, bring your hands down until they are straight in front of you at shoulder height.

Keep your shoulders wide.

Now relax your shoulders.

Bring your hands down to your sides.

4

5

6

aim

– To stretch and relax the neck muscles.

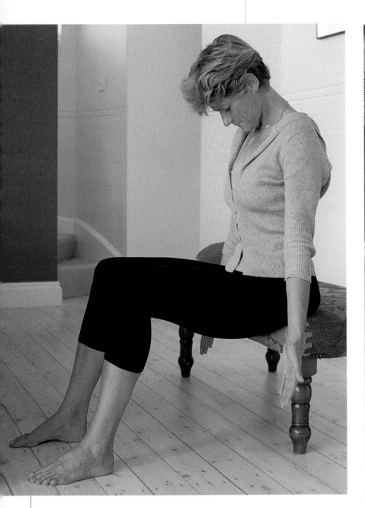

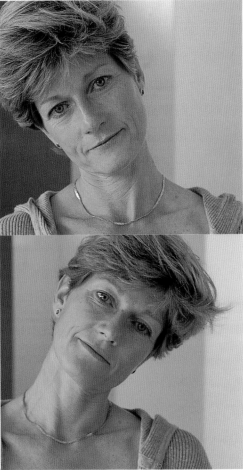

Sit on the edge of a chair or bed. Tuck your chin in towards your chest.

Allow yourself to melt like an ice cube from your chest and stomach muscles, letting the spine drop forwards.

Hold the position for **10–30 long, slow breaths**.

Repeat 1–3 times.

Sit on the edge of a chair or bed.

Drop your right ear towards your left shoulder as far as is comfortable.

Hold the position for **10–30 long, slow breaths.**

Repeat on the left side.

Repeat 1–3 times.

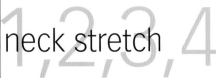

neck stretch

variation

aim

– To massage and stretch the
muscles of the feet.

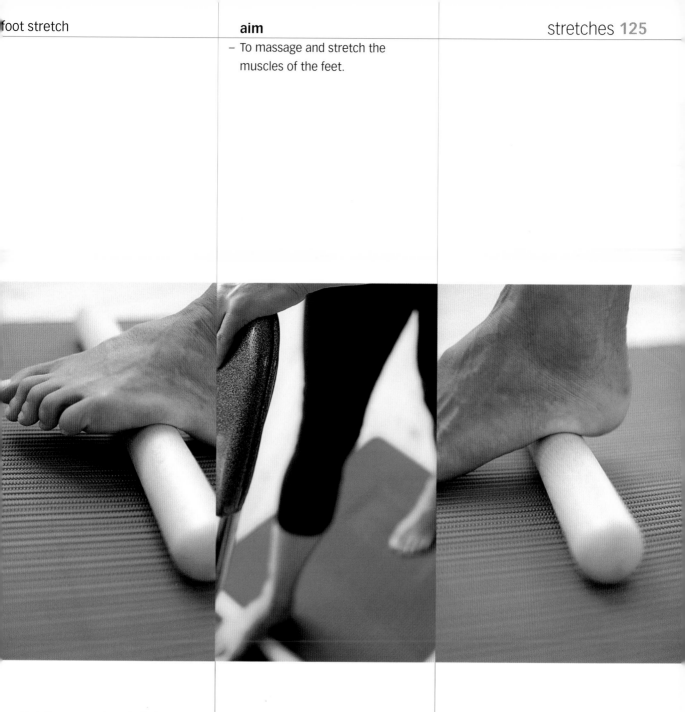

Holding onto the chair for
balance, place your toes on
the rolling pin, pushing firmly
down onto it.

Press the weight of your body
onto the rolling pin and slowly
roll the sole of your foot over it,
from your toes to your heel.

Now roll back again slowly
from your heel to your toes.

Repeat 6–10 times with
each foot.

1

2

3

foot stretch

aim

– To release tension in the jaw, which
  will help to relax the neck.

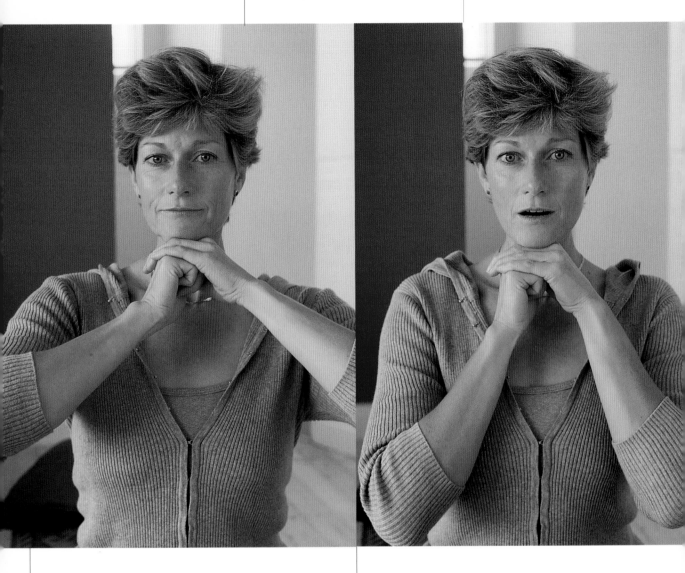

Make one hand into a fist and wrap your other
hand around it.

Rest your chin on your hands.

Open your mouth until the teeth are one finger-
width apart.

Keep your upper jaw still while pushing your
lower jaw into your hand creating active
resistance.

Hold for a count of 10.

1

jaw stretch 1

2

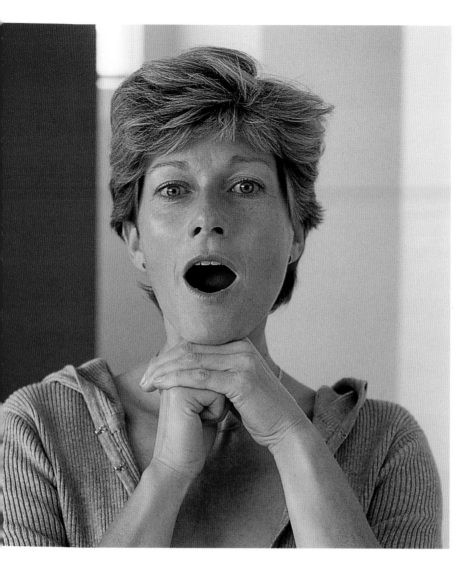

Repeat the Jaw Stretch with your mouth about 2 finger-widths apart.

Hold for a count of 10.

Repeat, this time with your mouth as wide as you can.

Hold for a count of 10.

variation

Acknowledgements in Source Order

Photo Credits

AKG, London 33 Top, 33 Centre

Kingston Museum & Heritage Service/Eadweard Muybridge Collection: Kingston Museum 13 Top Left, 32

All other photography Octopus Publishing Group Ltd./ Mark Winwood